# Of One Mind

*The Logic of Hypnosis*
*The Practice of Therapy*

Also by the author

*Completing Distinctions*
*Writing Between the Lines*

A Norton Professional Book

# Of One Mind

*The Logic of Hypnosis*
*The Practice of Therapy*

## Douglas Flemons, Ph.D.

W. W. Norton & Company
New York • London

For information about permission to reproduce
selections from this book, write to
Permissions, W. W. Norton & Company, Inc.,
500 Fifth Avenue, New York, NY 10110

Composition by York Graphic Services
Manufacturing by Haddon Craftsmen
Production manager: Leeann Graham

**Library of Congress Cataloging-in-Publication Data**

Flemons, Douglas G.
    Of one mind: the logic of hypnosis, the practice of therapy/Douglas Flemons.
        p.      cm.
    "A Norton professional book."
    Includes bibliographical references and index.
    **ISBN 0-393-70382-7**
    1. Hypnotism—Therapeutic use.    I. Title.
    RC495.F56        2001
    615.8'512—dc21        2001044250

W.W. Norton & Company, Inc., 500 Fifth Avenue, New York, N.Y. 10110
www.wwnorton.com

W.W. Norton & Company Ltd., Castle House, 75/76 Wells Street, London
W1T 3QT

1 2 3 4 5 6 7 8 9 0

To Shelley, Eric, and Jenna

# Contents

# Acknowledgments

Had it been just up to me, this book would have been finished years ago, around the completion time I'd originally projected. But fortunately, the book—long before it *was* a book, back when it was still just scraps of a manuscript—had a mind, and an agenda, of its own. The more I tried to hurry it along, the more it dug in its heals, demanding that I give the ideas a chance to form, develop, and interrelate. After some initial frustration and despair, I started listening to, and then respecting, its cautions. This changed our relationship, which in turn changed the writing. When the book and I got on the same page—when we became of one mind—the ideas, the words, starting coming, albeit slowly, ever so, always so, slowly.

The pace and process of the writing affected not only me. All the important people in the life of this book—my family, editor, friends, colleagues, students, and clients—exercised wonderful patience and support, offering me the necessary freedom to figure out what I was trying to say. For this I am deeply grateful.

Shelley Green, my wife and colleague, stuck with me from start to finish, reading drafts, offering on-the-spot, spot-on suggestions, and helping me keep my sense of humor when the ideas were playing hide and seek. Eric and Jenna, our sparkling children, provided me with daily doses of curiosity, mischief, and laughter. Lately they've been saying, "Daddy, are you thinkin' what we're thinkin'?" I'm thinkin' their question is a great description of hypnosis.

At the start of this little adventure, Susan Munro, my editor at Norton, asked me to write a twenty-word description of the book. In composing a response to this cogent request, I was able to distill an understanding that served as a compass when I felt most lost.[1] Throughout, I appreciated Susan's interest, trust, and minimalist style. Deborah Malmud, also at Norton, inherited me a couple of years ago when she was hired into Susan's position. Adapting herself to my production speed, she kindly facilitated my working with Susan until the end.

My clients generously invited me into their lives and minds, where they taught me much about hypnosis, therapy, and the art of improvisation. My students at Nova Southeastern University and the participants in my workshops peppered me with just the kind of questions necessary for me to hone my explanations and, in so doing, to discover what I was thinking.

I got some of my initial ideas down on paper in 1991, in response to an invitation by Ray and Dorothy Becvar to come to St. Louis and give a day-long workshop as part of their "Quiet Voices" series. Over the next year, my talk turned into a fifty-page paper that a couple of journal editors told me needed to be put on a starvation diet. I sent the manuscript to Jeff Zeig, who gave the opposite advice. Given that you're reading this, you already know to whom I listened. Frank Thomas helped me jumpstart what became Chapter 2 by asking me to contribute a chapter to his and Thorana Nelson's *Tales of Family Therapy*. In 1998, Rich Simon suggested I write something for what was then called the *Family Therapy Networker*. Working on that article helped me find and fine-tune the tone I had been seeking.

Michael O'Neill offered me a piece of his piece "Ontophony" to illustrate a point in Chapter 1. Sean Byrne provided some cultural consulting. Sandra Roscoe allowed me to use her dissertation research as a jumping-off point for Chapter 5.

Several people—family, friends, colleagues, and former and current students—helped me by reading drafts, offering inspiration, requesting consults or supervision on cases, giving me permission to write about them, helping transcribe tapes, and so on. I'm particularly grateful to Khawla Abu-Baker, Judy Adelson, Jennifer Albert, Carl Arrogante, Irma Barron, Roxanne Bamond, Ruchi Bhargava, Art Bochner and Carolyn Ellis, Martin Borthick, Tommie Boyd, Bill and LaClaire Brown, Lex and Dorey Brown, Chris Burnett, Bruce Butler, John Carney, Ofri Cohen, Melissa DeMeo, Dan Digatano, Alex Dominguez, Barry Duncan, Merle Etzkorn, Peter Fitzgerald, Suzanne Ferriss and Steve Alford, les Flemons (Bet, Don, Joyce, Ralph, Tom, Ward, and Wendy), Arlene Gordon and Richard Ryal, David Hale,

Fanya Jabovin-Monnay, Barbara Janus, Tom Kazo, Martha Laughlin and Kate Warner, Dee Lexandra, Paul Maione, Tom Mahan, Mike Moxley, Mary Naples, Debra Nixon, Michael O'Neill, Manny Perez-Campos, William Rambo, Sandra Roscoe and Stuart Horn, Jim Rudes, AnnaLynn Schooley, Dawn Shelton, Cindy Silitsky, Muriel Singer, Miriam Stern and Diego Arango, Debbie Swayman, D'Aun and Herb Tavenner, Kaisha Thomas, David Todtman, Elena Tragou, Helene Van Heden, Julio Vigil, and Kristin Wright.

Thanks, y'all!

# Preface

One of my master's students once asked me to confirm something she thought she'd figured out about me. She and I and several of her colleagues were sitting around, going over the cases we'd seen in the practicum I'd been supervising all semester. Reflecting on some ideas and suggestions I'd just offered, and thinking about some of my therapy sessions she had read about and watched, she said, "You weren't trained as a family therapist, were you?" I had specialized in family therapy in both my master's and doctoral programs, so I was curious to know how she'd arrived at her conclusion. "It's just," she replied with a tone of mild accusation and slight bewilderment, "you're so *different.*"

I'm unclear how the comment was intended, but I took it as a compliment. I doubt she would have sounded so disconcerted, though, had she known more about the work of other brief therapists—Haley (1990), Watzlawick, Weakland, and Fisch (1974), O'Hanlon and Wilk (1987), Combs and Freedman (1990), Keeney (1983), or de Shazer (1982)—or other hypnotherapists, such as Gilligan (1987) or Matthews (1985). I certainly part company with each of these authors on various issues, and each of them, in turn, probably wouldn't agree with everything I've said in this book. But, like all of them, I've been inspired and influenced by the systemic ideas of Gregory Bateson and the hypnotherapeutic innovations of Milton H. Erickson.

As a professor in a family therapy graduate program for the last twelve years, I've had the happy responsibility of offering, yearly, a doctoral seminar on the ideas of Bateson (I call it Thinking Systems) and another on hypnosis, primarily focused on the work of Erickson. The two classes couldn't be more different—in both format and content—but each is indispensable for the other. Erickson anecdotes crop up as we're talking about Bateson's notions of relational mind, and Bateson's ideas help frame and explicate Erickson's relational methods. Although each man has been dead over twenty years, the two of them have continued to chat through my classes and in my head, their conversation providing a counterpoint to the exchanges I have with my students, my supervisees, my clients, and myself. Yet, despite my debt to both men, this book isn't *about* either of them; rather, it offers my take on what hypnosis is and how it works and, following from this, it develops a host of ideas and suggestions for how you can effectively and creatively help your clients change.

In addition to teaching didactic courses, I provide ongoing live supervision of family therapy practicum teams. At last count, I had logged three thousand or so hours behind a one-way mirror, watching therapeutic interviews and doing my best to figure out what's helpful, what isn't, and why. I also maintain a private practice, in which I see people for hypnotherapy and brief therapy. I tell my supervisees stories about my work with my clients, and I tell my clients stories of my students' cases. Weaving through it all is my writing— the place where I can reflectively sort through my muddles and epiphanies, inventing ways of making sense of what I'm learning. This book is the result of such efforts.

As a therapist, supervisor, teacher, and writer, I'm committed to helping people take risks: to question their assumptions, to venture new ways of thinking and acting, to open themselves to new experiences. I will consider this book a success if you, too, find my ideas, stories, and suggestions *different*—different enough, at least, to inspire your taking a second look at your therapeutic habits and choices; different enough to help you freshly appreciate the curious logic of hypnosis, hypnotherapy, and brief therapy; different enough to bring forth your own and your clients' freedom and creativity.

# Introduction

The royal road to solving the mind-body problem involve[s] unraveling the mystery of hypnosis.

—*T. X. Barber*

What is required is precise talk about relations.

—*Gregory Bateson*

*"Poison," Joannie[1] moaned, tears of fear and pain wetting her face, "I have poison running through my veins. Poison, poison, . . . it hurts so bad, so bad."*

*Five months pregnant, Joannie had gone the previous week to her ob/gyn complaining of serious pain in her arms, pain that had been keeping her from sleeping and often reduced her to tears. Unable to find a physical explanation for her distress and not wanting to prescribe pain medication, the doctor had suggested she try hypnosis. And that's just what she had been doing—trying hypnosis with me in my office, accepting my invitation to enter trance—when the sensation of being poisoned overwhelmed her.*

In a moment, I'll tell you how I responded to Joannie's startling pronouncement, which will give you a taste of how I think and work, as well as a feel for what you can expect from the rest of the book. But first let me comment on my use of the word *trance* in my opening description. If, when you read it, you pegged me as a "special-state" theorist, then you have some unpegging to do. I agree with the critics who say that defining hypnosis as an altered state of consciousness is an exercise in tautological reasoning. Self-referential nonsense results when the "state" of hypnosis is used to explain the existence of hypnotic phenomena, which, in turn, are used to define the hypnotic state.

Thus, despite my fondness for the word *trance*—which I use for sound etymological and philosophical reasons (see Chapter 1 and the Glossary)—I don't consider hypnosis a special state. Rather, I view it as the creation and maintenance of a special *relationship,* a relationship that bridges the mind-body division, altering, while it continues, the everyday boundaries of the conscious "self."

If this doesn't yet make much sense, stay tuned. You'll have a much better handle on it by the end of Chapter 1, after I've teased apart the relational organization of mind and made clear the relational structure of negation, metaphor, and categorization. These ideas provide the necessary strands for me to weave a relational explanation of hypnosis and therapy: what hypnosis is and how and why it works; why your clients' efforts to banish or control their symptom exacerbate it; and how you can best facilitate therapeutic change.

As I point out in Chapter 1 and discuss further in Chapter 2, therapeutic change is, for me, a movement toward freedom, although not the sort our clients typically request. They, looking for a "cure," want freedom *from* their problem, but, given the relational nature of mind, we can only help them find freedom *in relation to* it.

In Chapter 2, I demonstrate that freedom is important in *all* the relationships relevant to your therapeutic work—not only the one between your clients and their problem,[2] but also in the relationships between your clients and you and between your clients and themselves. To be effective, you have to find ways not to be constrained by their requests or demands (see Chapter 4) and, concomitantly, not to let your thoughts and emotional responses constrain *them* (see Chapter 3).

Take Joannie, for instance. How do you suppose you'd react to her? Would her poison talk put you off? Unnerve you? In Chapter 3, I describe the importance of using your metaphoric imagination to get beyond seeing your clients as Other. By immersing yourself in their world, by imagining yourself as them, you can move from outsider to insider and, in so doing, begin inventing opportunities for change that fit the idiosyncratic logic and details of their experience.

*"Joannie," I said, "the poison hurts so bad. . . . How fortunate, then, that poisons have antidotes. Go ahead and let the antidote for this particular poison enter your arms and start to transform it. I don't know if the antidote will cause the poison to evaporate through your pores . . . or to drip out the*

*ends of your fingers . . . or to neutralize it in some other way. Let's let the antidote begin working and see how the poison changes."*

*Joannie's face relaxed a little and her tears stopped. After a few minutes, she whispered, "The poison's been dripping out my fingertips, but it won't completely drain out. It's pooled in the ends of my fingers."*

Some therapists might consider the poison's behavior to be a species of resistance—an obstacle to change that must be overcome. Chapter 4 presents an alternative view. I figure clients will always find themselves, at various times, needing to say *no* to me and/or to what I'm suggesting at the moment. Why shouldn't they reject what doesn't fit for them? I respect how their saying *no* helps to ensure their safety and define their integrity, so I don't try to overcome it. Instead, I adapt my position and alter my approach so as to render it *unnecessary.*

*"If the poison can pool in the fingertips of both hands," I speculated aloud, "it's certainly capable of becoming concentrated in the fingertips of just one of them. I wonder which?"*

Clients begin saying yes to the possibilities we offer when they stop finding it necessary to distinguish themselves from us and our ideas. This is a defining feature of hypnosis, where the connection between hypnotist and client renders their differences, for the duration of the trance, mostly irrelevant. The development of such interpersonal rapport makes possible an analogous intrapersonal shift. In Chapter 5, I use a transcript of a hypnosis session to illustrate what happens—and what becomes possible—when your clients stop experiencing themselves as distinct from their own experience, separate from their body, thoughts, memories, sensations, emotions. With their mind embodied and their body mindful, clients are in a position to discover the exhilaration and freedom (and sometimes weirdness) of not-consciously-dictated change.

*A few more minutes passed. "It's moved to the fingertips of my right hand."*

Now what would you do? Suggest that she use her left hand to squeeze the last vestiges of the poison out of her right fingers? Try to get the poison to leach into her fingernails and then get out a pair of clippers? See if a stronger dose of antidote would do the trick? Chapter 6 uses ideas first introduced in Chapters 1 and 2 to elaborate a way for you to think about and invite therapeutic change—creating, nurturing, and developing innovative possibilities for significant, and sometimes surprising, transformations.

*"Marvelous," I replied, "Isn't the homeopathic wisdom of your body amazing? For if your body is going to continue to manufacture the antidote to the poison, it is going to need to keep a little of the poison around to serve as a homeopathic catalyst, no? Can you check with the fingers of your right hand and see if it is okay for them to hold just enough poison for the ongoing manufacture of the antidote?"*

So why did I not try to get rid of those last drops of poison? I have no patience for the idea that clients somehow "need" their symptom, and I certainly wasn't trying to be perverse. Rather, my choice was determined by my appreciation of how symptoms arise, why they stick around, and how they go away. This appreciation, in turn, is based on my understanding of how hypnosis works. The logic of hypnosis lies at the heart of therapy. Once you grasp it, you'll find yourself orienting to problems—and to the process of doing something about them—in a significantly different way.

*After a long pause, Joannie said, "That will be okay."*

*"Realize that these fingers might experience some ongoing discomfort. They might be a little stiff, or a little cold, or a little uncomfortable at times. Are they willing to experience that—to serve as the site for the homeopathic manufacture of the antidote?"*

*Another long pause. "Yes."*

*Joannie's arm pain all but disappeared after this session. Her right fingers felt a little uncomfortable at times, but she was able to sleep well, and, for the rest of her pregnancy, she required no pain medication other than the occasional Tylenol.*

When you start thinking relationally about hypnosis and therapy, you'll be able to encounter your clients—whether individuals, couples, or families, and regardless of the particularities of their struggles—with respectful curiosity and mischievous anticipation. How will you, this time, invite them to connect with you, to connect with themselves, to connect with their problem? How will you invite relationships that protect your freedom to act and inspire your clients' freedom to change? Turn the page, and I'll offer you some ideas that later, when you're with your clients, you can bring alive in a way that fits for you and them.

# Of One Mind

*The Logic of Hypnosis*
*The Practice of Therapy*

My mind is not something confined inside me. A good deal of it is inside me. But a good deal of it is outside. It is in books. It is in notes. It is in my five fingers if I use them to count with, to do arithmetic with. . . . Well, now what happens when you and I talk? . . . Obviously all the things that I do, which are picked up by your perceptions, are a part of you. And things that you do, which are picked up by my perceptions, are a part of me. And there's an enormous overlap in our two minds. So that it is not unreasonable to speak of a "shared mind." This is not a miraculous phenomenon; it is a common-sense phenomenon.

—*Gregory Bateson*

The only reasonable excuse for adding another theory of hypnosis to the many which have been proposed is an entirely new approach to the problem.

—*Jay Haley*

# 1

# Hypnosis, Concordance, and the Self[1]

The antithesis *conscious/unconscious* probably does *not* hold the clue to further advance of psychological theory. It requires modification or reinterpretation in terms of more comprehensive and precise ideas.

—*Lancelot Law Whyte*

The mental world . . . has it roots in the twin facts of *distinction* and *classification.*

—*Gregory Bateson*

Whatever [a child's] first words actually seem to be saying, the first urgent message—to parents, sisters and brothers, visitors, strangers on the sidewalk, the family dog—is "Think with me." And, once begun, this becomes life's mission for almost all of us, surely all but the most unlucky. "Think with me" is what we really mean when we use the term *consciousness.*

—*Lewis Thomas*

I magine you're sitting in the recliner in my office, and let's say you
have asked me, and I have agreed, to invite you into hypnosis. You
have your doubts about whether anything will happen, what with all
the distracting noises down the hall, the thoughts swirling and racing
in your head, and your concern about "losing control." Despite your
reservations, you decide we should give it a shot, so I start talking.

As you sit back, resting your gaze there on the wall, . . . and now
on the floor, . . . moving your gaze to just the right place, while the
rest—. . . the phone out there ringing, . . . (until someone picks it
up), the voices out there murmuring (too low to pick up what they are
saying)—the rest *out there* can carry on with their busy-ness . . . while *in
here* . . . the gentle breeze from the air vent . . . the hum of the air con-
ditioner . . . the relief knowing someone else is out there to race around
and pick up the phone, while *in here,* now, we needn't be bothered.

How fast can your thoughts race? . . . Remember racing around
when you were four or five? . . . Racing here . . . to there, . . . racing so fast that everything seemed in slow motion . . . the way a tennis
player watches her opponent's backhand smash . . . sllloowwllyy zoom
across the net, . . . leaving an eternity for her body to move into just
the right position to respond? . . . Her body in a high speed, slow motion dance with her opponent and the ball. . . . What a luxury to race
so fast that you can keep up with yourself, . . . enter into a high speed
slow motion dance with your thoughts, . . . sensations, . . . perceptions, . . . with me, . . . with the crisp sharp walk of that person
walking down the hall out there. . . . A friend of mine, when he walks
with me, always stays a step or two ahead, regardless of whether I speed
up . . . or slow down. . . . He likes to stay ahead, just ahead, . . . as
we do our slow motion high speed dance down the street, . . . together, in step, him leading the way. . . .

Now at some point your eyelids may decide to close. . . . Your blinks may get longer . . . and longer, step by step, . . . or maybe, just out of the blue, they will just up and decide to close, all on their own, . . . when they decide they are good and ready. . . .

After a while, your eyes close, and, a little later, your arm responds to my suggestions for it to levitate.

And I wonder whether one of these hands here will stay slightly ahead of the other, . . . not moving down the street, of course, but rather up off your lap. . . . Which will be first to become enlightened about its ability to lift up? . . . Or do they already know how, so that the rising is simply a matter . . . of one or both getting the lead out? . . . Will one hand upstage the other? . . . Or encourage the other to downplay . . . its uplifting ability? . . . But will the other hand take the first one up on this suggestion, or choose, instead, to be the first one up? . . . Waiting, . . . up in the air about which will be second, . . . I wonder where and how the movement will first start? . . . In a finger? . . . Two fingers? A palm? . . . Your hands, too, may, at this moment, be up in the air . . . about which will be first . . . to be up in the air. Or perhaps they already know.

Your right hand lifts, in small little jerks, a foot or so off your lap, followed somewhat later by your left. I make some suggestions regarding loss of sensation, and you discover that your left arm, in particular, has become remarkably numb.

At the end of your appointment, you pepper me with questions:

What went on? Was this hypnosis? What *is* hypnosis, anyway? Was I in a trance? How could my arms levitate on their own? It felt like I had nothing to do with their rising up—did I? Did I do it or did you? How did my left arm lose its feeling? Why did our hour together feel like ten minutes? And what has this got to do with therapy?

You were right—your thoughts *do* race, don't they? Given what I observed and you described, I would say that, yes, you experienced hypnosis. Given how weird you felt when your arms were floating, you would probably agree with those hypnotists who consider hypnosis to be a special state of awareness or a unique state of consciousness. But I'd like to offer you another way of understanding what happened. Instead of regarding your experience in terms of your having entered a special *state,* I would describe it as the development of a special *relationship,* or, rather, two special relationships—one between you and me, and the other between you and yourself. In each, something odd happened to the boundaries of your "self," to the way you were *distinguishing* and *making sense* of who, what, and where "you" were. To explain this shift in your experience of yourself, I'd like to talk a bit about the business of *knowing,* about how you and I perceive and understand the world and our relationship to it.

## *Knowing*

Separating entities from their surroundings is what allows us to perceive them in the first place. In order to discern any "thing," we must distinguish that which we attend from that which we ignore.

—*Eviatar Zerubavel*

It is a cardinal precept of modern (structural) linguistics that signs don't have meaning in and of themselves, but by virtue of their occupying a distinctive place within the systematic network of contrasts and differences which make up any given language.

—*Christopher Norris*

Basically, there are two kinds of terms: terms that put things together, and terms that take things apart. Otherwise put, A can feel himself identified with B, or he can think of himself as dissociated from B. . . . Socrates' basic point about dialectic will continue to prevail; namely, there is composition, and there is division.

—*Kenneth Burke*

Sitting in my lap when she was nine months old, my daughter, Jenna, reached out, grabbed my watch off the table in front of us, and put it in her mouth. To manage this feat, she had to be able to distinguish the watch as an *object,* and, to do that, she had to differentiate it from the table. Of course, for her, the watch wasn't a *watch;* it was simply an *item-to-be-tasted.*

Contrast this with something my son, Eric, said at eighteen months. Pointing to the watch on his mother's wrist, Eric exclaimed, "clock!" He was not only *isolating* the object (against the background of the wrist), but he was also, in language, *categorizing* it, making a connection between it and the contraption on the wall of our kitchen.

To be able to put stuff in your mouth, you have to be able to *distinguish* it, and to do that, you have to be able to *separate* it from what it isn't. Then, to *make sense* of that stuff, to find it meaningful, you have to be able to *connect* it to or associate it with something else. This is how we think. We separate stuff out and we make connections between it and other stuff. These two activities—separating and connecting—are the warp and woof of all mindful activity (see Flemons, 1991). As such, they can help illuminate how hypnosis and therapy work.

## Separating

Since most, if not all, awareness involves discrimination, or
consciousness of a contrast or distinction, we shall provisionally
assume that conscious aspects of mental processes are distinctions.
                                          —*Lancelot Law Whyte*

The Cartesian "revolution" made the crucial absolutist and
analytical error (for us) of unjustifiably conferring a privileged
ontological status on entities ("substance") as opposed to
relationships. In spite of Aristotle, Hegel, and Marx, the truth that
entities do not create relationships so much as RELATIONSHIPS
CREATE ENTITIES was (and still remains) generally obscured.
                                          —*Anthony Wilden*

The viewing of the world in terms of *things* is a distortion supported
by language. . . . [T]he correct view of the world is in terms of the
dynamic relations which are the governors of growth.
                                          —*Gregory Bateson*

You see a tree against the sky, hear a siren through the drone of traffic, feel a cold current in a warm ocean, experience an epiphany out of confusion. Each time, you consider the thing you perceive to be a discrete object. Jeremy Hayward (1987) describes well the nature of such reification:

> The tendency to regard the world as being made up of separate entities, "things," having their own separate existence and identity and only accidentally related to other "things" is the most deep-rooted characteristic of human thought. We can call it the "fallacy of separate existence." (p. 226)

The fallacy is this: You, like old Rene Descartes, think of the world as a bunch of discrete selves, solitary individuals, detached perspectives, and independent entities. But, in fact, *nothing* in your awareness exists in isolation. Your seeing, hearing, feeling, and experiencing are dependent on the *relationship between* foreground and background, between what something *is* and what it *isn't*.

⌐‾‾‾‾‾‾⌐
**tree** / sky

⌐‾‾‾‾‾‾‾‾‾‾‾⌐
**siren** / traffic drone

⌐‾‾‾‾‾‾‾‾‾‾‾‾‾‾⌐
**cold current** / warm ocean

⌐‾‾‾‾‾‾‾‾‾⌐
**epiphany** / confusion

As Gregory Bateson (2000) used to say, you perceive *difference*.

Ironic, eh? To know something as an isolated thing, you have to draw a distinction, and the distinction creates a relationship. Your thing-thinking—your *thingking*—appears to be peopled with objects, but each of those entities is part of a *relationship*. Mind is fundamentally *relational*.

## SELF AND OTHER, MIND AND BODY

The self is a relation that relates itself to itself or is the relation's relating itself to itself in the relation; the self is not the relation but is the relation's relating itself to itself.

— *Søren Kierkegaard*

I have been reading your Descartes. Very interesting. "I think; therefore I am." He forgot to mention the other part. I'm sure he knew; he just forgot to mention, "I don't think; therefore, I'm not."

— *Katagiri Roshi* (via Natalie Goldberg)

The trouble is all in the knob at the top of our bodies. I'm not against the body or the head either: only the neck, which creates the illusion that they are separate.

—*Margaret Atwood*

Talk to most mental health workers, and they will tell you that dissociation is a sign of psychopathology (e.g., Lynn & Rhue, 1994).[2] Talk to a hypnotist such as Ernest Hilgard, the man responsible for the "neodissociation" theory of hypnosis, and you will be told that dissociation is an indicator, or even a determining factor, of the "hypnotic condition" (e.g., Hilgard, 1973). Talk to me, and I'll underscore dissociation as an essential characteristic of normal conscious knowing.[3]

In your everyday, walking around, negotiating-your-way-through-the-world state of awareness, you not only distinguish between those isolable things (objects, ideas, and so on) we were just talking about, but you also distinguish between them and *you*. If you are at all like me, your conscious self experiences itself as a kind of transcendent observer and director, separate from the world "out there." But it doesn't stop there.

Where do you locate your "I"? Where do you locate the conscious "I" who says, "My hand hurts"? Who thinks, "I hope she likes my idea"? Who fumes, "My anxiety is bugging the hell out of me"? I locate mine in my head. It's like I have a little homunculus up there, a little miniature "I"—an *i*—who draws a primal line between itself and everything else, including the rest of me.

Listen again to how you experience yourself:

"My hand hurts."

"I hope she likes my idea."

"My anxiety is bugging the hell out of me."

Your hand, idea, and anxiety are yours; they are part of who you are. But notice the sense of ownership implicit in your statements: "*my* hand," "*my* idea," "*my* anxiety." If your hand, idea, and anxiety are *yours,* if they *belong* to *you,* then they remain distinct *from* you, from the inner, insular *i* that remains distinct from *them.* Your connection with the rest of you—your body, your thoughts, your emotions—is made within the context of a separation, within the existential dissociation between owner and owned, between conscious knower and consciously known.

You/me, I/you, mind/body, self/experience—when we differentiate one from the other, we end up not with independent *entities* but with interdependent *relata*. Despite what you and I consciously assume, despite what our dissociative self awareness—our *thingking*—inclines us to believe, you and I act, live, hope, fear, write, speak, discern, suffer, delight, and remember *in relationship*.

## NEGATION

A child, visiting, had been admonished by his mother not to ask for things, but to wait until they were offered to him. He was standing before a bowl of bananas, looking at them hungrily. The hostess asked him what he was doing. He answered: "I am *not* eating a banana."

—*Kenneth Burke*

Negation, as the dialectical logicians recognize, and as Freud himself came to recognize, . . . is a dialectical or ambivalent phenomenon, containing always a distorted affirmation of what is officially denied.

—*Norman O. Brown*

He drove the thought away angrily. It returned and sat outside his skull. Like a dog.

—*Arundhati Roy*

One morning when Jenna was two and a half, I overheard her talking to an odd-looking vehicle in Eric's toy-car collection. Holding the flat-bed conveyance as if it were a baby, she was attempting to lovingly explain to it what or who it was by defining what or who it *wasn't*. "You're not a car," she said, "not a truck, not Mommy, not Daddy, not Brother." Finally, she concluded, "You aren't anything."

Negation is a primary tool for dissociative *thingking*. We use it in language to create separations: to differentiate (this is not that), clarify (this does not mean that), hope (this does not have to be that), challenge (this is not acceptable), deny (this is not true), reverse a position (this is no longer true), establish individual identity (I am not you), and so on. But such separations can never be "pure." Whenever you use negation to separate something from something it isn't, you forge a relationship—a *separated connection*—between the two. Jenna's negations didn't create a positive stand-alone identity for her vehicle; it became a not-car, a not-truck, a not-Mommy, a not-Daddy, a not-Brother.

We often try to apply a kind of conscious, dissociative logic to our problems, identifying something we hate or fear (be it anxiety, drinking behavior, the tendency to explode in anger, or whatever), attaching *no* to it, and then treating the negated thing as an isolable possibility, a discrete non-entity (a potential *no-thing*), capable, by virtue of its negated identity, of being flushed out of existence. We can only fail at such attempts; as I explained earlier, mindful (perceptual and languaged) acts of separation connect, and thus we will always find ourselves experientially *connected* to that from which we purposefully *separate*.

Think about what happens when you set out to forget something you cannot bear to remember: The damned memory returns to haunt you. The poet Brian Fawcett (1981, p. 52) caught the heart of such dilemmas most poignantly:

> *How many times I've wanted*
> *to forget you, forget*
>
> *the things you told me in the dark*
> *sweet scents of your body, the bouquet*
>
> *of enchantment in each flower*
> *we knew together*
>
> *elusive and shortlived, overpowered*
> *by the empty habits*
>
> *that keep life*
> *from flowering. Yet*
>
> *each time I've tried*
> *to forget you*
>
> *groggy with sleep or too much drink,*
> *there is the memory of wildflowers*
>
> *and the faintest rueful scent of you*
> *blossoms in the stalest air*

When such negations fail to achieve the desired end, you can always then attempt, as a Zen master once proposed (cited in Watzlawick, 1984, p. 169), to negate the negation:

> *To think*
> *that I will no longer think of you*
> *is still thinking of you.*
> *Let me then try*
>
> *not to think*
> *that I will no longer think of you.*

But your second-order *no* ties you to your first, which, in turn, ties you to whatever you wish to escape. Even negated negation offers no easy freedom, no simple way out—it merely serves up a double dose of dissociative logic.

When you say or think *no*, such as when you say, "I will not think of her," you create a distinction:

**not thinking of her** / thinking of her

As a result, the thing you want to get rid of (in this case, "thinking of her") sticks around as the necessary complement to your negation ("not thinking of her"). As Bert and Ernie confirmed during a scientific experiment on *Sesame Street*,[4] attempting to separate from something via negation creates an inadvertent connection:

> Bert, dressed in pajamas and a nightcap, is ready to turn in for the night when he notices Ernie setting up a drum kit next to the bed. Ernie explains that they are about to conduct a scientific experiment, the first step of which requires the posing of a question.
>
> ERNIE: The question is, "Will you be able to fall asleep if I *don't* play these drums?" . . . And the only way to find out the answer to that question is to do an experiment. I will sit here and *not* play the drums and you try to go to sleep. . . .
>
> Bert considers the experiment (and Ernie) a little loopy, but, amused and a little perplexed, he agrees to participate.

BERT: It's a great experiment. You sit there not playing the drums and I'll just get into bed and we'll see what happens. Hello dreamland! Here comes Bert! . . .

Bert snuggles under the covers and tries to get comfortable, but before long, he sits up and worries aloud that Ernie will start banging the drums as soon as he falls asleep.

ERNIE: No Bert! I'm *not going to play the drums*. That's what the experiment is.

Reassured, Bert attempts again to settle into sleep, but he keeps tossing and turning, tossing and turning. Finally, he explodes:

BERT: That's it! I can't sleep! I can't sleep! I can't! I can't!

ERNIE: You can't sleep with me sitting here not playing my drums, Bert?

BERT: No! I can't! I tried, Ernie! Believe me, I tried. But I can't! I can't!

ERNIE: Then my experiment is over! I have discovered the answer to my question! You can't sleep if I sit here, not playing my drums!

Ernie's experiment demonstrates that you can't create a positive mood—such as "sleepy comfort"—by negating a negative mood: You can't settle into relaxed tranquility by striving to be not-tense. Attaching *no* to unwanted thoughts, feelings, memories, behaviors, and so on never eliminates them from your experience; rather, it ensures their continued presence and importance. The effort to negate creates a dissociative relationship, a separated connection between a person and the problem he or she despises. The feared, the hated, the not-wanted—whatever you attempt to negate sits outside your skull, like a dog. Or next to your bed, like a silent drummer.

Consider, for example, a woman who diligently tries to manage thoughts of killing herself by actively not thinking of suicide; or a man, unable to leave his house without waves of panic, who tells himself over and over not to feel afraid; or another man who adamantly refuses to walk in the park near his home as a means of controlling his desire to expose himself there.

**not thinking of suicide** / thinking of suicide
**not panicking** / panicking
**not exposing** / exposing

Suicide, panic, and the possibility of exposure loom ever larger in these people's respective lives, in spite, indeed in part because of, their (and others') attempts to respond dissociatively to their defined problems, to use negation to banish what they don't want.

Most clients want you to help them negate their symptom. But given the relational structure of language and thought, any effort in this direction risks further entrenching the very thing they so desperately want eradicated. Instead of helping your clients *dissociate from* a symptom, you would be better off helping them *associate with* it or with something else instead. In the process, you will have an opportunity to invite the symptom to change or transform or, as it loses significance, to ease away into relative obscurity and irrelevance. I'll be discussing this approach to problems in great detail in Chapter 6, but before it'll make much sense, you'll need to understand how connections work.

## Connecting

Only connect!

> —*E. M. Forster*

Look for connections!

> —*Miss Frizzle*

Without context, there is no meaning.

> —*Gregory Bateson*

You make perceptual connections all the time. Your eye clusters dots on a page into distinct objects

        •   •      •   •

           •     •   •

and your ear clusters notes into patterned wholes, or melodies.[5]

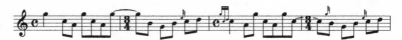

You also make connections in language, sometimes via categories, other times via metaphor. A category connects things in terms of a shared, named attribute: A watch and a clock are both *timepieces;* you and I are both *therapists;* disgust and joy are both *emotions.* A metaphor also creates a link between things, but rather than classifying the association in terms of an abstract entity, it collapses one thing into the other, defining *two* as *one:* "time is money"; "a poem is a pheasant";[6] "love is a river."

Let's look at categories first.

## CATEGORIES

Classification implies a relation of resemblance between members of the same class, and one of dissimilarity between members of different classes.

*—Jean Piaget*

An understanding of how we categorize is central to any understanding of how we think and how we function, and therefore central to an understanding of what makes us human.

*—George Lakoff*

Things become meaningful only when placed in some category.

*—Eviatar Zerubavel*

What is the last book you read? A novel? A biography? A dictionary? The category *book* connects a variety of such objects, as well as sacred tomes; how-to and self-help manuals; religious, philosophical, and political treatises; collections of recipes, poems, essays, photographs. In establishing a link between these items, the term *book* defines them as a group, thereby distinguishing them from other associational clusters, such as airplanes, vegetables, and lampshades.

The members of a category are like the members of a sports team—they tend to stick together. If Joseph Heller's *Catch 22* is lying on your kitchen counter next to the zucchini you plan to fry for dinner, the physical proximity between the two won't be enough to prompt you to associate them. Instead, you will make sense of the rectangular object by classifying it as a member of the category that also includes the dictionary in your living room and the science fiction you read as a teenager. And you will make sense of the green oblong object by classifying it as a member of the category that also includes the eggplant in your fridge and the onion you forgot to buy at the store.

To make sense of something, you must categorize it, defining it in terms of its similarity to other things. As the saying goes, blood is thicker than water; likewise, intra-category relationships are thicker than extra-category relationships. The "blood" relationship between *Catch 22* and the *Oxford English Dictionary* is thicker than the "water" relationship between the novel and the zucchini sitting next to it. Between the book and the vegetable is a *gap of insignificance*.

An interplay of meaning operates between a category and its members, between a connected whole and its separated parts. You change the meaning of *book* when you classify something new (say, a stapled assemblage of comic strips) as a member of the category, and, conversely, you alter the meaning of a thing when you classify it differently, when you contextualize it via different associations or give it a different name. This is the theoretical rationale for the therapeutic practice of "reframing" (i.e., recategorizing or reclassifying) the component parts of a pattern. Because meaning is dependent on context, and because categories contextualize experience, reclassifying something can have profound consequences for people. I'll give you a clinical illustration of this in a moment, but first let me tell you a little story about crying and bears.

At fifteen or sixteen months, Eric enjoyed imitating the sounds made by various animals, but he derived the most pleasure from making the ferocious, guttural "Roarrrr!" of the bear. One day when I was holding him, he got upset about something, and I heard him take a big breath. I knew he was about let out a frustrated howl, so I quickly whispered in his ear, "What sound does a bear make?" The "Arrggroarrrr!" that followed began as an expression of his angry mood, but it was *also* an answer to my question. Eric's eyes started to dance, and by the time his lungs were empty, he was feeling playful and happy, his mood transformed by his experience of his recategorized wail.

My wife, Shelley Green, once supervised a family therapy case (Green, 1994) in which a similar recategorization was achieved. An eleven-year-old girl and her siblings were brought to Shelley's therapy team by their mother, who was worried about her daughter

Melanie's inability to measure up to the two sisters with whom she shared the classification *triplet*. Megan and Mindy were thin and pretty and did well in school; Melanie was significantly heavier, did poorly in most of her subjects, was fighting with her sisters and with her peers at school, and had been diagnosed as depressed. The triplets all wore identical clothes (though different sizes), but this didn't keep strangers who saw the three of them together from considering Megan and Mindy as twins and Melanie as just their sister. Such reactions proved most discouraging for everyone. All members of the family tried to help Melanie remain a true triplet, but everyone failed to keep her from failing. The family understood the girls to be fraternal triplets (from three separate eggs), but they all treated and had expectations of them as if they were identical. In fact, though, the girls were not all equally different (i.e., fraternal) triplets. Shelley and her team of therapists figured out and helped the family understand that Melanie differed biologically from her two sisters—she was, in fact, a fraternal triplet to identical twins. The therapists suggested that another, older, sister in the family might be able to help her figure out how to be "just a sister" to Megan and Mindy.

With her unique place in the family finally acknowledged and accepted, Melanie blossomed. Her mood brightened, her grades improved, and she made new friends. During a subsequent session and a longer-term follow-up, she continued to show and talk about the positive changes that had transpired as a result of her new identity.

The case dramatically illustrates how context—the connection between things—imparts meaning: When Melanie's relationship to her fellow triplets changed, so did Melanie. It also demonstrates how you can create comfortable separations by encouraging new connections. Two years before coming to see Shelley and her team, the family had seen a psychologist, who had urged the triplets to stop dressing alike. But trying *not* to be triplets had, of course, reinforced triplethood—the girls, following those earlier sessions, had returned to dressing identically, and Melanie had continued to flounder. By focusing on pulling the girls apart, the psychologist had inadvertently tied them together. He didn't understand how negation works.

Shelley and the therapists on her team took a different tack. Rather than urging Melanie to "try hard *not* to be a triplet," they suggested that she consult with her older sister about being a sister to twins.

They thus offered the possibility that the family could consider Melanie a *sister-of-twins-and-other-siblings* rather than a *triplet*. Creating a stronger association between Melanie and her older sister effectively made her triplet connection with Megan and Mindy less important. The separation wasn't created via an imposed negation (*"Don't* be a triplet") but, rather, by way of a connection elsewhere ("You and your older sister have more in common than you thought"). Such association-generated gaps of insignificance I call *connected separations*. My story of Eric's roar provides another example of how they work. Had I admonished Eric not to cry as he took his big breath, my attempted negation of his crankiness would have highlighted it, perhaps inspiring him to become still more upset. By giving him, instead, the opportunity to hear his wail as the sound of a bear growling, I helped him transport himself into the realm of play, and his displeasure slipped away unnoticed. The connection between him and the bear created a connected separation between him and his bad mood.

Let me give you one other example. Remember my session with Joannie, the one I described in the Introduction? When she found that the poison in her arms wasn't going to completely drip out the ends of her fingers, I categorized the lingering amount as a homeopathic catalyst. This connected her discomfort to the process of healing and recovery, thereby creating a connected separation, a gap of insignificance, between the sensation in her fingers and the pain she had been experiencing in her arms. Had I tried to negate the poison ("do whatever you need to do to make that remaining poison disappear—keep at it till there is no poison left"), her pain would have, I'm sure, given her the silent drummer treatment.

### METAPHOR

All knowledge is ultimately rooted in metaphorical (or analogical) modes of perception and thought.

—*David Leary*

Metaphor is not just a matter of language, that is, of mere words. . . . On the contrary, human *thought processes* are largely metaphorical. . . . The human conceptual system is metaphorically structured and defined.

—*George Lakoff and Mark Johnson*

Metaphor is not just pretty poetry, it is not either good or bad logic, but is in fact the logic upon which the biological world has been built, the main characteristic and organizing glue of [the] world of mental process.

—*Gregory Bateson*

Metaphor is the inverse of negation. If metaphor asserts, "Love is a river," negation protests, "Love is *not* a river." Both declarations are ironic—though, predictably, in opposite ways. Negation denies any connection between love and rivers—"love is *not* a river"—but the denial undermines itself: The *not* that separates love and rivers connects them. Metaphor proclaims the oneness of love and rivers—"love *is* a river"—but this claim, too, undermines itself: The assertion of oneness can't be made without keeping distinct, and thus separate, the two things being joined.

Still, just as negation is primarily dissociative in form, metaphor (from the Greek *meta-*, over + *pherein,* to carry: to carry over) is primarily associative. When you think metaphorically,[7] that is, when you give priority to the connection between the distinct things you are associating, you may find yourself not taking much, if any, notice of the boundaries separating them. Transference is a good example.

If you respond to me as if I were someone else—your father, a former lover, your firstgrade teacher—then I would be willing to describe your metaphoric connecting of me and this other person as transference. For you, the pattern of our relationship will echo in some significant way (be a metaphor of) the pattern of your relationship with this other person, but you may well not be aware of the connection. This has much to do with the business of conscious discernment I talked about earlier. Unless you isolate a relationship, a connection, as an object of your scrutiny, concretizing it in language and thought as a demarcated thing, it will hover at the periphery of your awareness. A not-noticed relationship remains, by definition, unconscious—not consciously discerned. Thus, your metaphoric connection of me and the other person will remain outside your ken until you or someone else isolates it as a thing, as something that can be consciously noticed and considered.

Shelley and I once saw a dating couple who had had an upsetting interaction during sex (see Flemons & Green, 1998). The man believed there to be something wrong with the woman because she, in the middle of what they both considered consensual lovemaking, had suddenly started screaming at and hitting him. Just prior to this point, the man had begun playfully holding the woman's wrists above her head. This was a new position for them, but it had been mutually agreed upon, so they were both initially confused as to why she had suddenly become, as they described it to themselves (and later to us), so violent. After a cooling down time, the two of them began talking about what had happened, whereupon the woman recalled that, when she was raped some twenty years earlier, the rapist had held her down in the same body position as her boyfriend. This resulted in her reacting to the boyfriend in terms of her relationship with the rapist, even though the sexual encounter with the boyfriend did not resemble the rape in any other way. Her associating the two experiences was a metaphoric connection that operated outside of her conscious awareness until after she and her boyfriend started talking.

Metaphoric thought accounts not only for your making not-recognized associations between things or people "out there," but also for your ability to lose track of the boundary separating yourself—your insular *i*—from your body, from other people, from your environment. And when that boundary becomes, for a time, irrelevant, your experience of yourself and your surroundings changes significantly. This is what happens when you lose yourself in a movie, get caught up in a novel, get transported by a piece of music, lose your head in a new relationship, feel an empathic outpouring for another person, or get carried away dancing. In each of these experiences, as in hypnosis, you drop your Descartes impersonation—you no longer experience yourself as if your *i* were the director of your thoughts and the owner of your body.

Remember the expression for when you and another person are in close agreement over some issue? We say the two of you are *of one mind*. As "you" stop defining yourself in contradistinction to whomever or whatever you aren't, your *i* disappears, and you and that other become *of one mind*. For example, when I'm watching a film, my attention floats somewhere between my seat and the screen. When the protagonist meets with trouble, my heart quickens, and when he or she encounters tragedy, my eyes tear up. The distinction between "me" and the protagonist becomes unimportant, and thus imperceptible, as

I allow myself to experience the metaphoric relationship, "I am the protagonist."

This happens to me, for varying lengths of time, every time I see an excellent film. Sit me down, though, in front of a poorly made or poorly acted movie, or one that, for whatever reason, fails to capture my interest, and I will stay constantly aware of myself and my surroundings. When I'm critical of what I'm seeing on the screen, I watch in my usual conscious-of-myself-being-conscious mode, distinguishing myself from the film and the characters in it. At such times, I am eminently distractable.

I am to movies what my mother is to novels. When she is reading, you can pretty much forget trying to get her attention. Three, four, five times you will need to call her name before she will finally look up from the page. While she is absorbed in the narrative in front of her, her otherwise acute sense of hearing is significantly dampened, she seldom is aware of herself turning the pages, she loses track of time, and she doesn't notice minor aches and pains. This too is an instance of metaphoric thought process: She gets carried along in the story as if the events described were happening to *her*.

One more family story: My dad's dad—affectionately known as "Grump"—had a rule in his house. Whenever he put on a recording of classical music, everyone had to sit still and listen. Watching his face, you could tell he was inside the music. I'm sure he never had the explicit thought, "I am the violins," "I am the french horns," "I am the symphony," but his experience was certainly structured metaphorically: The distinction between Grump and the music became, for the duration of the symphony, unimportant. And his listening rule helped him ensure that nothing would disengage him from his music.

Such connections also happen to people actively involved in physical activity. As Wayne Gretsky skated around and between the players on an opposing team, he wasn't distinguishing himself from his arms and hands, himself from his legs and feet, himself from his stick, himself from his skates, himself from the puck. Similarly, as Michael Jordan out-maneuvered his opponents, he wasn't separating himself from his arms and hands, himself from his legs and feet and shoes, himself from the basketball. The knowing of athletes extends into and loops back from their bodies and their surroundings.

Something analogous happens with musicians. Take, for instance, the playing of jazz pianist Bill Evans:

> He sat sort of erect at the piano, and he'd start to play. And pretty soon his eyes would close, and his upper body would gradually start to lower itself, until finally his nose would be about an inch away from the keyboard. It was as if he were abandoning his body to his muse—as if the body evaporated, and there was some direct connection between his mind and the piano itself. It was not a put-on, and it couldn't have been comfortable.
>
> When he'd finish playing, he was like a person being revived from some reverie. He'd been so immersed in whatever that process was, and then the applause would bring him back. He'd sit up, and blink his eyes—like he was coming to. It was very strange. (Larry Bunker, as cited in Nolan, 1996)

Evans surely wasn't playing from a detached place in his head, demarcating self from hands, hands from keyboard, keyboard from notes, playing from hearing, hearing from hands. For the duration of his time inside a tune, Evans would have found such distinctions irrelevant.

During such times of metaphoric experience, you don't stop drawing distinctions. You see and hear the action on the movie screen, you read the words in front of you, you discern different instruments and melodies and harmonies, you differentiate your opponents and teammates on the rink or court, and, if you are a jazz musician, you distinguish chords and modes as you carve an improvised line. But the distinguishing self—the *i* that is distinguishing this and that *out there*—stops distinguishing *itself,* stops setting itself apart. It experiences itself as *a part of* knowing rather than *apart from* the known,[8] becoming of one mind with something other than itself—the body, another person, a tool or instrument of play, and so on.

Ever stood in an empty concrete stairwell and found and held the particular note that creates an echo? Ever sung in a large choir, surrounded by people holding the same note as you? When you are producing the same note that is enveloping you, the boundary that differentiates inside and outside is, for a moment, canceled out. Your physical awareness of yourself as separate and distinct disappears, and you feel a sense of oneness with your surroundings and/or the other singers. This is how metaphoric knowing affects your *i,* and it is how your self-defining boundary changes within the experience of hypnotic trance.

## *Hypnosis*

Most great ideas come to people in transit.

—*Evan S. Connell*

The mind is inherently embodied.

—*George Lakoff* and *Mark Johnson*

The etymology of the word *trance* is identical to that of *transit* (*trans,* across + *ire,* to go), which the O.E.D. defines as "the action or fact of passing across or through." If you think of hypnosis as the *active crossing* of the boundary between your *i* and the rest of you, then *trance* becomes a useful term for characterizing the perception of that boundary becoming, for a period of time, indistinct. The word *hypnosis,* though, is another story.

Coined by James Braid, a Scottish surgeon, in the 1840s, *hypnosis* comes from the Greek *hupnos,* meaning *sleep.* As EEGs have shown, the phenomenon the word names has nothing to do with sleep (Bowers, 1976, p. 130), save for the outward appearance of some of the people experiencing it. Based on the ideas I have outlined, a far better word would be *concordance,* the Latin root of which—*concorde*—the O.E.D. defines as "of one mind" (from *con,* together + *cord-,* heart: *concorda-re,* to be of one mind). Instead of a *hypnotist,* we would call me a *concordist,* and, as such, my job would be to concord with you and to help you concord with yourself.

Unfortunately, I'm a hundred-and-fifty or more years too late to introduce a substitute term for *hypnosis.* Braid himself suggested that *monoideism* (having one dominant mental idea) was an improvement over his earlier coinage, but the new word never caught on. Resigned to using a bankrupt word, I will tell you a story that has kept me from throwing it out altogether.

When he was about two years old, Eric loved the *Curious George* books. In one of the stories, George, a little monkey, starts crying after falling off his bicycle. Reading the passage of this misadventure,

I would often take on George's frustration and pain, pretending to sob as I croaked out the sentences. Eric would look at me with a mixture of humor and concern, firmly pat my face, and demand, "No Daddy, wake up!" He knew I wasn't asleep, but he had, at the time, no other way of saying, "No Daddy, let go of your metaphoric connection to George; return to your normal Daddy-who-distinguishes-himself-from-storybook-characters way of talking!" Hypnosis isn't sleep, but had Eric (at age two) seen you immersed in your hypnotic experience, had he watched your metaphoric connection to me and to yourself, he might well have patted your face and told you to "wake up"—to, as it were, return to your "normal" nonparticipatory way of knowing.

During my "trance talk" with you, I invited metaphoric knowing by speaking in time with your breathing, by arranging "word clusters" to coincide with your exhalations. And I practiced what the Ericksonians call *utilization:* By mentioning the ringing phone, the murmuring voices, and the footsteps just as they occurred, I linked my words to your perceptions, folding whatever was going on "out there" into our connection "in here" (see Erickson, 1980). Possible distractions inspired images and stories. I associated your racing thoughts with your racing as a child, and then, with the description of the tennis player, introduced the notion that you could race in slow motion. If time is relative, your zippy thinking could thus facilitate, rather than hinder, your hypnotic experience. The person walking down the hall became a sound effect for a story of my not getting flustered by my friend always staying a step or two ahead of me. You, analogously, could then relax into not having to slow yourself down to my speed, not having to worry about giving me control. We could be together *and* you could still take the lead.

To the degree that I connected with your experience, the boundary between us

$$X/Y$$

became unimportant, and you and I became of one mind:

$$X \Longleftrightarrow Y$$
$$\Downarrow$$
$$X = Y$$

Although I was attempting to create this sort of metaphoric connection between us, I should underscore that such efforts can, and should, never fully succeed. The professional boundary separating you from me must obviously remain in place for you to remain safe and for me to remain ethical. But within the context of our distinctive positions, I did what I could to render temporarily unimportant (for you) any of the other innumerable differences between us.

Some hypnosis theorists would say that as I talked, you became more "suggestible." Others would say that your "suggestibility" is a stable trait, a "hypnotizability" capacity that distinguishes you from people who can't be hypnotized and aren't suggestible. I'm not fond of either characterization, as each places "suggestibility" inside of you as a localizable *thing*. If what happens in hypnosis has to do with changes in *relationship*—changes in the relationship between you and me and between you and yourself—then we shouldn't waste our time looking *inside* of you for an explanation of what goes on.

When you argue with an opponent, you each negate the other's position, defining your respective selves and ideas as separate and distinct. But when you brainstorm with a friend, you lose track of who is responsible for what idea. Your connection allows you to experience the relationship metaphorically: I am you; you are me. At such times, you attend less to who says what than to what *fits* for you.

As you and I got in sync in our hypnosis session, you became comfortable trying on my suggestions. When they fit, you, like anyone engaged metaphorically with another, weren't concerned with determining the *source* of the ideas. You didn't find it necessary, for the most part, to distinguish yourself from me or your ideas from mine; and your body, similarly, didn't separate itself from the suggestions that it, too, could engage in thoughtful behavior. I view this not as suggestibility but as unanimity (*unus,* one + *animus,* mind). We— you and I, and you and yourself—were, as it were, unanimous. We concorded.

The ideas and images I offered you were designed to help you experience being of one mind with *yourself*, to help you experience a metaphoric connection between your knowing-self and your known-self, thus making the boundary between them irrelevant. As you wondered with me when your eyelids would decide on their own to close, and as we speculated about which hand would first find itself rising to the occasion, you were accepting the possibility that know-ing could take place on both sides of your mind-body split. With the closing of your eyes and the raising of your hands, you quit distin-guishing yourself as an insular knowing *i*, separate from me, separate from the passage of time, separate from your thoughts, emotions, sensations, and perceptions. This marked your movement into hyp-nosis, into concordance.

When Evan S. Connell said that "most great ideas come to people *in transit,*" he was referring to people moving physically through space, but his comment applies equally well to people *in trance,* to people moving mindfully across the boundary between self and other, between *i* and body. The associational movement of trance facilitates the generation and receipt of great ideas. I'll have more to say about this in Chapter 5, where I discuss hypnosis and hypnotherapy in greater depth.

You felt like you weren't responsible for closing your eyes or lifting your hands, no? Nor did you feel like you were "making" your hand numb or purposefully losing track of time. You were right: "you" weren't doing these things—or, at least, your *i* wasn't. With your *i* not cutting itself off from everything, it couldn't take ownership of and responsibility for the movements of your body or the changes in sen-sation and time orientation. Instead of your knowing being bottled up inside your head, it crossed the boundaries between you and me and you and your body. I guess we could say it got "distributed." This felt to you like your body had a mind of its own (and the way I phrased my suggestions implied that it did). But it didn't. *We*—you and I; you and your body—had a mind of *our* own. You were simply experienc-ing consciousness in keeping with what the word originally meant—to know (*scio*) together (*con*) (see L. Thomas, 1990).

Our and your one-mindedness also allowed you to experience something else. Released from the dissociative control of your *i,* a couple of eyes and arms and a hand and a sense of time were able to feel *free,* free to move and change in unpredictable ways. The possi-bility for such freedom—relational freedom—is central not only to hypnosis, but also to therapeutic change. When you can find ways for your clients to stop dissociating from their symptom, when you cre-ate a one-mindedness, a concordance, that includes you, your clients, and whatever they've been trying to banish, you allow the symptom the relational freedom to move and change in curious and surprising ways. As you saw with Joannie, once she was able to stop pushing her pain away, it was free to transform independently of her conscious intent. But this way of orienting to cases is also relevant beyond the borders of hypnotherapy. In the next chapter (and then throughout the rest of the book), I show how the notion of relational freedom can be used to shape your orientation to clients, their problems, and therapeutic change, regardless of whether you are using hypnosis.

# 2

# ational Freedom

> e relationship between the thing and some
> n the thing and you, or part of you, never the
> thing itself. You live in a world that's only made of relationships.
>
> —*Gregory Bateson*

**Relation**. . . . **3**. . . . . That feature or attribute of things which is involved in considering them in comparison or contrast with each other.

**Relational**. . . . **2**. Of, belonging to, or characterized by relation in general.

**Freedom**. . . . **4**. The state of being able to act without hindrance or restraint, liberty of action. **8**. Of action, activity, etc.: Ease, facility, absence of encumbrance. **11**. The state of not being affected by (a defect, disadvantage, etc.)

> —*Oxford English Dictionary*

As part of my teaching responsibilities, I supervise a small team of family therapy graduate students in a weekly six-hour practicum. At the beginning of each semester, I pester my team members to articulate their understanding of therapeutic change, to say how they make sense of it and how they think it happens: "What the hell is therapeutic change?" I ask them, "And what is your piece of the action?" After they lay out their premises, I detail mine. In this chapter, I tell you what I tell them.

Do you remember the time when Winnie the Pooh, Rabbit, and Piglet got lost in the woods? Again and again, they tried to find a way out, a way home, but every time they set off, their efforts to escape kept returning them to their point of departure, to "a small sand-pit on the top of the Forest" (Milne, 1985, p. 263). Pooh Bear became "rather tired of that sand-pit, and suspected it of following them about, because whichever direction they started in, they always ended up at it" (p. 263). Finally, Pooh reasoned that if going in search of his home resulted in their returning to the sand-pit, then going in search of the sand-pit should result in their finding their way home. The approach worked, and soon the trio achieved their freedom.

In Chapter 1, I talked about the relational nature of perception and language, about how nothing exists (from the Latin *ex-*, out + *sistere*, to stand: to stand out) in isolation. You and I and our clients experience this connectedness every time we try to negate some kind of sand-pit, some aspect of ourselves or another person with which we are uncomfortable. If our psychological and social worlds were truly composed of isolable *things*, we could easily obliterate objects to which we objected. But we live in a web of *relationships*, so whenever we try to cut off or push away something we identify as Other (whether inside or outside ourselves), our attempted separation forges a connection—a *separated connection*. The more we treat a problem as an entity to be controlled, eliminated, or shunned, the more we sand-pit-ize it, and the more it follows us about. Caught in the weave of relational thought, we become entangled by our efforts to free ourselves.

As a (hypno-/brief/family) therapist, I consider myself a kind of *disentanglement consultant*. Rather than focusing on clients' problems per se (as would befit someone wishing to nail down proper DSM-IV diagnoses), I attend to people's *relationships to* their problems. Asking how my clients have been handling what's vexing them, I listen for ways their efforts at severing the relationship may have tightened it into knots.[1] I think of therapy as a process of loosening and untying, rather than cutting through, such tangles.

In their sand-pit adventure, Pooh and his friends stumbled across an important relational truth, perhaps *the* truth about therapeutic change: The only way you can rid yourself of something you don't want is to find a way for it to become unimportant to you. But in a relational world, such an accomplishment can be very tricky, indeed. Purposefully separating yourself from something that troubles you—trying to make it insignificant, make it go away, make yourself forget or ignore it—only heightens its significance in your life. Pooh and company found an excellent solution to this dilemma. Instead of trying to escape from the sand-pit, they went *in search* of it, and this, for good relational reasons, allowed them to leave it behind.

By about fourteen months of age, my daughter, Jenna, had developed both a desire for her brother's possessions *and* a sense of entitlement. She didn't have too many words at her disposal, but her face had no trouble conveying what she was thinking whenever she grabbed one of Eric's toy cars: "I like this little sporty number, *and I deserve it*. In fact, let's just agree that it is now mine. If you don't want me to scream, I suggest you not even *think* about taking it away from me." Eric, who was five and a half at the time, *did* think about rescuing his toy from Jenna's tenacious grip, but he knew enough about toddler psychology not to cause a ruckus. He would either let her hold the car until she lost interest and dropped it, or he would divert her attention with some other toy—something that squeaked or was brightly colored or that flapped around when he waved it in front of

her. As Jenna became fascinated by and reached for this new entice-
ment, Eric could casually slip the car out of her hand.

The challenge for Pooh, Rabbit, and Piglet was to separate themselves from something they didn't want; the challenge for Eric was
the opposite: He had to separate his sister from something she *did*
want. But in both instances, the challenge was met, the problem was
solved, by the making of a connection. Pooh and his friends set off
with the intent of *finding,* rather than escaping, the sand-pit. Eric
recognized that when his sister became comfortably connected to his
car, when she could hold it, knowing she wasn't in imminent danger
of having it taken away from her, she relaxed her grip on it. And
when she became attracted—connected—to a different toy, his car
became insignificant. Once a connection is made, a *connected separation,* a relaxed letting go, becomes possible.

I don't know if Eric will choose a career in psychotherapy when he
becomes, as he used to put it, a grown-up man, but between his learning Pooh-Bear logic[2] and learning how to respond to Jenna's gripping
fascination with his toys, he already has the basics down. A therapist's
job is to facilitate change in the relationship between clients and their
problems, to help turn separated connections—engendered by efforts
at negation—into connected separations. To manage this successfully,
you have to remember that the freedom you have to offer is always *relational.* You can only help people begin to find freedom *in,* not *out of,*
relationship to their problems. When clients connect with whatever is
troubling them, when they stop treating it as Other, they are freed
from its stranglehold. By relaxing their banishment efforts, they allow
the trouble to become less troubling—to stick around in a more inviting atmosphere or to amble away, perhaps returning intermittently
for a brief reunion, perhaps forgetting to come back altogether.

Wouldn't it be great if you could just explain these notions to your
clients in their first session and they would go off and incorporate
them into their lives? But if effecting therapeutic change were that
simple, self-help manuals would render therapists obsolete. It's not
that didactic information can't be helpful, but I've never had much
success just giving clients good advice. For an idea to take hold, for a
possibility to become illuminated, for a pathway to be opened, it
helps for people to be able to *experience* it firsthand, to embrace it as
part of who they are. When they examine something intellectually,

subjecting it to their critical intelligence, they necessarily keep it separate, at arm's length. I prefer to offer an idea—a possibility for change—in a way that allows clients to embrace it with their metaphoric, participatory knowing. As Milton Erickson understood so well, this is why hypnosis can be helpful: It facilitates *relational change* rather than *rational understanding*.[3]

Given, then, that therapy involves more than the dispensing of good Ann Landers's advice, how *do* you help free up the relationship between clients and their problems? Certainly, my primary focus is on this question, and the primary purpose of this book is to answer it. But just as no *thing* stands alone, so, too, no *relationship* changes in a vacuum. You can't introduce relational freedom into the separated connection between clients and their problem (see Chapter 6) without also attending to (and often facilitating change in) a variety of other relationships, including the one between you and the clients (Chapters 3 and 4) and between clients and themselves (Chapter 5). Before starting to tease apart these relationships, I'd like to first describe a case that offers a sense of how they all entwine.[4]

Having heard of my hypnosis practice through a mutual friend, Alec called one morning to ask whether I could help make his father eat again. His dad, Mac, was seventy-four and dying of cancer. Following an operation three months earlier to remove a tumor from the base of his spine, Mac had all but stopped eating, complaining that he couldn't swallow without a great deal of discomfort. He had contracted thrush while in the hospital, but it had cleared up, and an endoscopy and other tests had revealed no physical cause for the pain in his throat or for his inability to eat. Although the doctors had found no tumors in this part of his body, Mac couldn't help but wonder whether the cancer had spread.

X-rays had revealed lesions on Mac's ribs, and chemotherapy had been ordered. But Mac hated the side effects of the chemo, and he didn't wish to prolong his dying, so he had decided to discontinue treatment. He also had decided to quit taking medication for his dangerously low blood pressure, as well as the antidepressants and appetite stimulants that had been prescribed. He continued to take a painkiller every four hours for the "hot spots" on his spine and ribs; unfortunately, it made him sleepy all of the time. His oncologist gave him six months to two years to live.

Each day Mac managed to sip half a cup of coffee and a glass of root beer, and he could get down an eight-ounce cup of blueberry yogurt, but that was his limit. The doctors were concerned about dehydration and the physical complications resulting from Mac's diet—he had lost thirty-five pounds since the operation. Every day Mac's wife, Hanna, cooked him tantalizing meals and chided him to at least taste what she had made, but his throat refused to cooperate, so he had no choice but to decline.

I told Alec when he called that I couldn't and wouldn't try to make his dad eat, but I would certainly meet with the family and see what, if anything, could be done. Mac was too weak to come into my office, so I went out to his and Hanna's home. Laura, their daughter, happened to be in town visiting, and Alec and his brother Jack were also available. I stayed two and a half hours that first visit; Mac joined the conversation for about an hour, after which he got fatigued and needed to lie down. He believed his wife and children were making too much of a fuss about his not eating. They accused him of giving up, of not trying, but, he said, such was not the case. He would eat if he could, but he couldn't. For whatever reason, his throat wouldn't open up, and he found it too upsetting to try to force anything down, so why, he demanded, didn't they all just back off?

Everyone agreed that Mac had always been the head of the household. All of them had a stubborn streak, but Dad, as Jack put it, was "Chief Billy Goat." He was a fiercely independent man who had encouraged the same in his children. In fact, he was irritated that Laura was flying in too often to see him.

"There's no reason for it," he grumbled, "I'm not about to croak yet. When I get close, okay, why not, but it's stupid for her to be spending all this money now."

Laura, of course, stubbornly refused to stay away, and she and her brother Jack lent their voices to Hanna's effort to convince Mac to be more reasonable about taking care of himself. Since he couldn't swallow, his health was deteriorating quickly, so they wanted him to agree to intravenous feeding or a feeding tube. He thought their suggestion ridiculous.

"This isn't a life anymore. What's the point? I feel like a nothing—why should I prolong this? For what? I've had a good life, and now I'm ready to die. End of story."

Tears filled Laura's eyes as she angrily denounced Mac as a quitter. "All my life you've pushed me to try. If I came to you for comfort, you told me not to be weak, to get back on my feet and keep fighting. So now it's your turn, and you just want to quit."

Hanna joined in. "The doctors say you could have two more years. But you're starving yourself to death. They say you've stopped eating because you're depressed. But you won't take the pills they gave you. They say there is nothing wrong with your throat. If you would just *try* to eat. Why can't you *try?*"

"I *have* tried goddamn it! If I could eat, I would, but I can't. My throat doesn't work, okay? After the first swallow, forget about it—it closes up. And anyway, I'm not hungry."

Alec seemed to be the only person who wasn't battling with Mac. He wanted his dad to enjoy his last days, but he wasn't pushing him. I wondered what would happen if others took the same approach. I asked the family many questions, but I think the most relevant one for them, the one that turned the discussion in a new direction, had to do with whether any of them could tell the difference between quitting and acceptance. I wondered how long before death arrived they would deem it appropriate for Mac to stop fighting. "If the doctors had said to you that Mac had only weeks, rather than months or a few years to live, would you consider his stopping the chemo and the medications a sign of depression and giving up hope, or evidence of his strength, his ability to stare death in the eye without flinching?"

Most of the family members agreed that if he had only a few months left, not fighting would be a sign of strength and acceptance. But what if, they asked, he still had a couple of years? Then his not eating and not fighting could only be seen as the actions of a quitter. So what was he, strong or weak? It all depended on how much time he had left. "What if," I asked, "Mac's body knows something that the doctor's don't? What if it is telling him that it is time to start preparing for death?"

Mac had to go lie down at this point. He was exhausted, and he wanted a cigarette. I continued the conversation with his children and, when she returned from settling Mac into bed, with Hanna. They told me that Mac had the disturbing habit of not calling for help when he needed to go to the bathroom. He would pull himself

out of bed and wobble across his bedroom by himself, despite the fact
that with his blood pressure so low, he could easily faint and, given
how frail he was, fall and break a hip. This didn't sound, I suggested,
like the action of a broken, depressed man, but rather that of a proud
and stubbornly independent one. If he had given up, why was he able
to keep all of them at bay so effectively? None of them had been able
to convince him to budge an inch on any of the decisions he had
made. I wondered aloud if the frustration and anger they all felt was
a measure of just how strong and stubborn Mac still was.

I asked if this self-reliant man had ever compromised on anything
that mattered to him. All concurred: "Absolutely not!" They all, at
various times in their lives, had gone head to head with him, and he
had always stood his ground. Chief Billy Goat. Not that he wasn't
sensitive and caring, they assured me—his and Hanna's marriage had
been one of equals, and he often had made changes in response to her
suggestions. But if push came to shove, no one was a match for him.
It was ironic, I suggested, that if they *were* successful at convincing
him to eat, it would be because he had lost the strength to fight back.
It thus made sense, given Mac's signature stubbornness, that the only
way he was likely to begin eating again—if he ever did—would be if
it were *his* idea. The family agreed.

I reflected with them on how difficult it would be for each of them
not to cajole Mac to eat. They loved him dearly, and if they were to
stop fighting with him over food, it could very well feel, at least at
first, that *they* were giving up, that *they* were contributing to his early
death. This was a very real risk. What if, when they stopped pushing,
Mac simply relaxed into the decision he had already made? Would
they then feel like collaborators? However, it seemed to me, I said,
that Mac would only begin fighting for his life, if he did so at all,
when he was given the freedom to do it for himself. If his wife and
children wanted to find out whether or not he could begin eating
again, they would have to let it be his discovery. This would also help
him to save face: Would it not be easier for a proud man to begin eating again because he had discovered his throat had somehow myste-
riously figured out how to work again, rather than because he had
been forced into it by his family?

Hanna agreed to continue cooking tantalizing foods, but not to directly encourage Mac to try them. She would let the aromas do their

own convincing, and she would ensure that, if he felt the urge to sample something, it would be available. The children, too, would provide their father with the opportunity to discover on his own whether or not food would be something he could enjoy again before he died. I reassured them that I would show the same respect for Mac as they did, and thus I would do nothing to "make" him eat. I would be willing, however, to explore with him whether it was possible for his throat to find a different way of working.

When I returned a week later, Laura had flown back home, and Alec and Jack were at work. Hanna met me at the door. Before ushering me into Mac's room, she told me that she had been making food for him, but with the attitude that "if he eats it, fine, and if he doesn't, fine." She realized that she had been angry much of the time, and that their arguments over food had gotten them both upset. This past week they had both been much happier.

I then met alone with Mac. We talked about cancer and death. I told him about my run-in with cancer a couple of years earlier: It was so strange to realize that my tumor had been growing for a long time without my having had any clue what was going on. In response, he told me a story about touring an army hospital ward during WW II. The colonel who had shown him around told him, "Mac, you can never tell how sick someone is by looking at him. That first guy you saw looked good, but he isn't going to last long, and the one who looked like he was on his last legs isn't nearly as sick as he thinks he is."

"Right," I said, "and you don't know if the new pains you are feeling are from new tumors, or from the healing process following your operation." Pain from healing can be a lot more tolerable than pain from something that is slowly killing you. I went on to tell him stories about how some people are able to feel sensations that aren't attached to anything physical (such as phantom limb pain), while others (such as mothers who manage to have pain-free childbirths) are able to do the reverse. In so doing, I was indirectly introducing the idea that the sensations he was experiencing could be unhooked from their physical source.[5] This laid the foundation for the hypnotic diminishment of his pain and the freeing up of his throat to work again.

Mac reiterated that he wasn't afraid of death but *was* afraid of dying too slowly. We talked about whether not eating would hasten the process. He told me that he really wouldn't mind eating if his throat allowed it. We agreed that he would talk to his oncologist about whether he would recommend hypnosis—if he did, we would meet for a subsequent appointment. I then walked him through the various ways he might find himself able to eat again, if that were to become possible. I didn't formally invite him into concordance, but I offered my ideas in a way that appealed not only to his understanding, but also to his body's experience:

> Your body has been on a long fast, and I'm not sure, if a reawakening of your ability to eat becomes possible, how it will come about. Hypnosis might be helpful, but you may notice changes in your eating and drinking even before we meet to do that, or even if we never get around to your going into a trance. If your ability to swallow changes, and whether that happens before hypnosis, after hypnosis, or without hypnosis, it could come about in a whole variety of different ways. There is no predicting just how such a thing might occur, just how a person's fast is brought to a satisfactory completion. I don't have any idea how your ability to take in and enjoy food and drink would be reawakened. . . .
>
> It could be that you start finding the aromas wafting out of the kitchen becoming interesting again. Your appetite may not change, you may still not, at this point, be able to swallow anything other than root beer and yogurt, but your sense of smell may become sharpened, your appreciation of smells heightened. . . .
>
> Or you may hear your stomach gurgling and suddenly realize you smell bacon frying. Or you may first notice the sizzling and only then notice the complementary gurgling. . . .
>
> Then again, the first sign may well not be a heightened sensitivity to the smells of bread baking or steak grilling. And you may continue not to be interested in the sounds associated with cooking—with the sound of a spoon stirring batter in a glass bowl, or of the clanging of a frying pan, or of popcorn popping. Ever been in a movie and eaten the popcorn without quite knowing that you were doing it? It may be that you are sitting at the table talking with Hanna and, without realizing it, you start munching on something on the table. You might not even know you've been eating until you see an odd look, a look of surprise in Hanna's eyes. . . .
>
> So too, you might simply find yourself *thinking* about food—thinking about it at odd times, or about odd foods at mealtimes, or odd foods at

odd times, like when pregnant women get it in their heads that pickles and chocolate ice cream are a perfect combination. . . .

It could be that you don't start thinking about food, or start eating it with that automatic enjoyment of someone watching a movie, or get intrigued with the sounds or aromas of cooking, but you just start feeling hungry. Maybe you'll be lying in here and you'll just, out of the blue, remember some special meal from your past. Perhaps it will be a romantic meal with Hanna, a birthday party when you were little, your first hot dog at a baseball game, the first good meal you had when you got out of the army. . . .

Or maybe you will just notice some subtle change that happens when you swallow your saliva, some small, almost imperceptible shift in how it feels to swallow, something that suggests to you that swallowing something other than blueberry yogurt is now possible. Perhaps you'll just decide, out of the blue, that you're interested in peach yogurt, or vanilla, or some other flavor. Your appetite may not change, but your interest in some sort of variation of flavor may be the first sign of something different. . . .[6]

I don't know what will be the first sign that your body is ready to swallow something different, and I don't know how it will come about, but if you decide to have another appointment, I'll be interested in what happens. It will be important for you to take care, though, because breaking a fast takes time and patience. You won't want to overburden your digestive system. . . .

Hanna called me a few days later and told me that Mac wanted to schedule another appointment. His doctor had told him that he could have anywhere from one month to ten years to live, so Mac figured hypnosis was worth a shot. When I arrived at their house, Hanna told me that soon after I left the last time, Mac suggested that she wheel him around the neighborhood in his wheelchair. He hadn't been outside, except to go to doctor's appointments, since his operation, and he had consistently refused to go for strolls with her when she had suggested it. They had gone out a number of times since. She also mentioned that Alec's wife, who hadn't seen Mac for a few weeks, had been over to visit and couldn't believe how upbeat her father-in-law had become.

I went into the bedroom. Mac told me he had been surprised the night before when he found himself enjoying a cup of chicken noodle soup and some crackers. A few days earlier he had tried, unsuccessfully, to eat a sweet potato, but he did pretty well with the brisket and gravy. He didn't understand how his throat had managed, the last three nights, to swallow something as dry and hard as pretzels, but he had enjoyed eating them, along with some ice cream.

At this point, I invited Mac into concordance with me, his surroundings, and himself, and I told him a number of stories that related to eating, swallowing, relaxing, body learning, changes in body sensation (for pain management), ending fasts, and so on. One of the stories had to do with how a friend of mine, a plumber, had managed, in a way that I didn't understand, to unplug a clogged drain in my house. Now I could put anything down it. Once he had finished clearing the pipe, my friend broke the news that he was moving soon, and he invited me out for breakfast the following week. We met and ate and reminisced about the times we had shared and what we had learned from one another. My friend's way of saying good-bye—the sharing of a meal and memories—had meant a lot to me. He told me he had been having many such breakfasts, saying good-bye to each of us who mattered to him.[7]

When we finished hypnosis, Mac said, "That was soft." His family didn't call for another appointment. I learned through our mutual friend that over the next six weeks, Mac was able to enjoy eating once again with Hanna, and that the family was warmed by his turnaround. He then began to decline, and a month later he died, after a short stay in hospice.

Alec told me a year or two after his dad's death that he and Mac had had some meaningful talks in those last weeks. Mac, a man whose rough-hewn exterior had sometimes kept people he loved at a distance, had had the time and strength to "get a grip on things," to rethink and reevaluate his life and his choices, and to say what he felt to those who could listen. When death came, Mac took his time chewing, and then he swallowed it whole. He held on until the day *after* Hanna's birthday— a last testament, in Alec's view, to his love for his wife.

Had I agreed, when Alec first called me, to use hypnosis to try to *make* Mac eat again, I would have found myself in the same position as those who loved him, creating a separated connection between the two of us by rejecting his throat's rejection of sustenance. Butting heads with Chief Billy Goat, I would surely have lost. But I also would have failed had I ignored what was going on between Mac and his wife and kids. How could his throat relax into changing when its curious behavior was under such impassioned attack from his family members? Without freedom in the relationship between Mac and these important others, freedom in the relationship between his throat and food and drink would have been difficult, if not impossible, to achieve.

Thus, before entertaining the possibility with Mac of his throat becoming open to change, I first helped Hanna and her kids recategorize their understanding of Mac's behavior, allowing them to consider his not eating as a sign of legitimate strength rather than as illegitimate weakness. By shifting from condemnation to acceptance, the family transformed their separated connection with Mac into a connected separation: They gave him permission to die. And by stopping trying to stop his throat from stopping food and drink, they gave it the freedom necessary to do something different.

Once the shift in the relationship between the family and Mac's throat had been shifted, I could then talk with Mac and get his take on dying. Had he told me that he welcomed his inability to eat and drink as an opportunity to die more quickly, I would have respected his throat's way of facilitating his decline, and I would have advised his family that there was nothing I could do. I made it clear to Mac that I had no investment in his lasting any longer than he wanted to, regardless of what his family might wish. He appreciated my respect, and he relaxed into knowing that we were of one mind on matters of living and dying. Once he knew I wasn't going to try to *make* him do *anything,* he clarified that he wouldn't mind enjoying eating and drinking again. This gave me permission to suggest possibilities for reconnecting to smells, ideas, flavors, memories, sensations, body processes, and so on. From there, it was a matter of his body figuring out a personal, face-saving way of bringing his fast to a satisfactory end, of letting go of its constriction.

Faced with a separated connection in some therapy-relevant relationship, you, as a disentanglement consultant, need to know how to respond so as to invite connections and connected separations. In the next two chapters, I talk about how to do just that in the relationship between you and your clients.

# 3

# Your Relationship with Clients

I think that's one of the great pleasures of being a human being—
that you can extend yourself, get outside yourself and identify with
somebody who appears to have nothing whatsoever to do with you.

*—Russell Banks*

Le coeur a ses raisons que la raison ne connaît point.
(The heart has reasons which the reason does not at all perceive.)

*—Blaise Pascal* (via Gregory Bateson)

We cannot step beyond metaphor. It is our only means of relating,
of connecting.

*—Donald F. Miller*

I conducted my first family therapy session during my second semester in a master's program in counseling psychology. At the request of a guidance counselor, I had been seeing, in individual sessions,
a bored and angry thirteen-year-old boy, Nick, who was failing his
classes and alienating his teachers. Nick wasn't interested in seeing me,
and I didn't have a clue how to talk with him, so I decided to invite his
mother, Helen, in for a joint session. I had recently watched some
videotapes of Virginia Satir working her experiential magic with es-
tranged families, and I thought perhaps I could wave a similar wand.

Helen and Nick arrived on time for their 7:00 p.m. appointment,
an hour after my supervisor had gone home for the evening. I began
the session by asking Helen what she thought was going on with her
son. She said that his father, Nick, Sr., was a no-good, dead-beat ma-
nipulator, and her son was blind and stupid: Not only did he look up
to his poor excuse for a father, but he was also following faithfully in
his footsteps. Nick shot her a withering look and told her to shut up.
Helen responded, loudly, that he was *never* to speak to her that way.
He repeated himself, and an argument ensued.

With my anxiety rising in direct proportion to Nick and Helen's
volume and intensity, I could think of no other questions to ask. Obviously, it was time for Satir to come to the rescue. I got in the middle of their escalating fight and asked them to turn their chairs so
they were facing each other. "Why?" Helen asked, with a note of in-
credulity and suspicion in her voice. I swallowed hard. Satir's clients
on the videotapes hadn't second-guessed her; they had simply followed her directives.

"Looking into each other's eyes should help you communicate
better."

"That's stupid!" muttered Nick, not moving his chair.

Helen agreed completely: "We already tried that with our last therapist. It was a total waste of time. Don't tell me I got off work early just so you could ask me to make a fool of myself. You're going to have to do better than that."

Mother and son grew less furious with each other as they joined in their dismissal of me and my stupid suggestion. "Why are you angry at me?" I huffed, relieved I wasn't (as Satir would have put it) placating their blaming stance, "I'm only trying to help you!"

By mutual consent, and without anyone resorting to blows, we decided to end the session early. Nick and his mother, more aligned (at least momentarily) than when they came in, left, convinced I was an incompetent therapist. I, shaken and chagrined, watched them go, convinced they were unsuitable clients.

Had I been able to talk with Nick and Helen about the stupidity of my request, about my wasting Nick's time in our earlier sessions, about their disgust with the string of professional non-helpers who had been suggesting nonsense, I probably could have turned our talk back to their relationship and their desire to change it. But my defensive anger at their dismissal of me cut short any such possibility. I pulled away, viewing them as strangers and myself as an outsider to their strange and unsettling behavior. I needed to find a way inside their "culture," inside their family, to connect with them as people, but I didn't know how.

In this chapter, I talk about how to avoid bungling as badly as I did with Helen and Nick—about how to move from an outsider to an insider, how to understand your clients' dilemmas, how to communicate your appreciation of your clients' situation, how to offer ideas that fit with their experience, and how to offer opportunities for change.

## When You Feel Like an Outsider

My practicum supervision of family therapy students is mostly "live"—while one of the students interviews a couple or family in the therapy room, the other practicum team members and I observe the session from behind a one-way mirror. Twelve years of such supervision has taught me how difficult it can be for therapists to get beyond viewing clients as Other, as strangers with strange habits and stranger ideas. Again and again I have seen my students (mostly, but not always, when they're sitting behind the mirror) react to clients with fear, pity, anger, boredom, amusement, repulsion, condescension, or professional "remove."[1] Such separated connections hold clients at bay, undermining the possibilities for therapeutic change. How can you and your clients tickle each other's imaginations if you're keeping them at arm's length? You can't think therapeutically as an outsider or with someone you consider an outsider. Allow me, then, to offer some ideas for how to become an insider.

## Acknowledge Your Estrangement

During my first few years of supervising, I became most impatient when behind-the-mirror team members would chuckle, groan, or mutter. More than once I accused a bemused or judgmental student of being lazy, of not thinking and acting like a therapist. My finger-wagging no doubt encouraged my team members to offer more politically correct comments and questions, at least when I was within earshot, but I doubt my admonishments helped them transform their negative assessments of their clients. I, myself, had once refused to work with a client whom I considered Other, and the experience made such a lasting impression on me, you'd think I'd have been better able to appreciate my students' reactions.

A wiry man with mirrored sunglasses had walked into a clinic where I was working, looking for a therapist. His wife had just taken their children and left him yet again, and he didn't know where they were. She had told him she would never return if he didn't get some therapy, so he guessed he would give it a try. Could I help him? I invited him into one of the therapy rooms to talk for a while. Although he left his sunglasses on, I did my best, at first, to connect with him. I didn't get too far—just enough to get scared.

Asked about what had been happening and what he wanted, he told me he was sick and tired of his wife walking out on him. Where did she get off thinking she could just up and leave whenever she felt like it? He hadn't even hit her that hard. He figured she needed to be taught a lesson. When she got around to coming back he was going to slap some sense into her. She'd pulled this running away shit one too many times and needed to know that she couldn't keep treating him this way. He wanted her, and he wanted his kids. There would be no more leaving. I asked how he could be sure of that. The next time she tried to leave, he said, he and his gun would make sure it was her last.

I've talked to many people about their hate and jealousy and despair, about their feeling crazy and terrified and hopeless, but no one else has managed to give me chills. This man wasn't asking for help to change; he was reporting a plan of action that left me afraid for his wife and children, and also for me. If his only hope of getting his wife back was to go to therapy, how would he react if I refused to work with him? And what would he do later when he found out that I had warned her of his intentions? Was he carrying his gun? Would he return? My fear would have dissipated had I found a way to appreciate his desperation, but I couldn't do that. His cold rage scared the hell out of me.

Fear, like anger and disgust, freezes curiosity and cements the other as Other. I told the man I had a problem. "If I see you for therapy," I said, "and you tell your wife about it, she may decide it is worth it to try again with you. But then if she does come back, she's going to get beat up. And then if the therapy is good enough to get her to return to you but not good enough to keep her from walking out again, you'll shoot her. That's too big a risk for me. I don't want to be a part of someone's dying."

He leaned toward me and whispered, "Don't worry, no one will ever know I was here. I won't tell nobody. Not even the cops. They'll never get it out of me."

I thanked him for his vow of silence but said that even if the cops never found out about me, I would feel horrible, thinking I was somehow responsible for his wife's getting hurt or killed. "And speaking of the cops," I continued, "do you know what they make me do? Any time I hear that someone might get hurt or killed, those goddamn cops make me warn the person. If I don't, I'll lose my license. So that puts you in a crummy place. Not only do I have to tell you that I can't work with you, but the cops make me warn your wife that her life is in danger." I thought this news might incense him, but, given he knew where to find me, I wanted him to hear it from me rather than his wife. He didn't appear overly bothered. After ending the session, I called a friend who worked at the local Women in Distress, and she passed on the warning. I never saw him again.

I considered my fear of this man to be legitimate, so I was comfortable with my decision to refuse his request for therapy. But a few years later when my first supervisees were reacting to our practicum clients with similar estrangement, I reproached them, telling them, in effect, not to feel what they were feeling. Considering *their* reactions to be *il*legitimate, I cast them as Other for their casting clients as Other.

### Kindle Your Curiosity

I figured out the beginnings of a better approach while supervising the work of a therapist who met with families in their homes.[2] One case in particular troubled him greatly. A mother and her teenaged son fought endlessly about the ways the boy was "messing up," and the mother wanted help in permanently placing him in some sort of facility. The therapist, a man in his early twenties, had, a few years earlier as a teenager, engaged in similar if not more daring activities than those of the son and, hence, identified quite easily with him. In fact, it was so natural for him to adopt the perspective of the boy that he had trouble letting go of it when talking with the mother. Like the son, he disliked her intensely. All she did all day, he lamented to me, was watch television, smoke cigarettes, and complain. Nothing the therapist said budged the mother from her conviction that her son was unmanageable and needed to be out of her house. And nothing I said as a supervisor budged the therapist from his dismissal of the mother. He had decided it was the mother, not the son, who needed institutionalization.

During our third supervision meeting, I stumbled across a useful idea for how the therapist could connect with his client. Remembering that he was an avid lover of movies who dreamed of directing documentaries, I suggested that he go on his next home visit not as a therapist, but as a filmmaker. "Assume," I said, "you have decided to make a documentary of this mother. Before bringing in the cameras, you need to find out everything you can about her life, so you can decide what scenes you will want to shoot. Go and interview her in preparation for the filming." His interest piqued, he agreed. When he returned for supervision the following week, he animatedly told me what a fascinating and wise woman his client had turned out to be. The two of them had spent a few delightful hours together chatting without the son present, and, in the course of their conversation, the therapist had developed a significant respect for the choices she had made and was currently making. This was the beginning of some productive sessions, where mother, son, and therapist worked together on successfully finding a time-limited placement for the boy at a sheriff's ranch. Rather than condemning the mother and attempting to shield the son from her, the therapist was able to be helpful not only in preparing both of them for the son's leaving, but also for his return— a possibility the mother hadn't previously considered.

By assuming the identity of a filmmaker as he interviewed his client, the therapist was able to let his curiosity get the better of his biases. Curiosity is a wonderful antidote for estrangement, for it pulls you across any self-Other boundaries you've imposed.

### Practice Seeing and Feeling Double[3]

I once supervised a case involving a family who had been terrorized by the children's father. The effects of the man's beatings and threats continued to send shock waves through the lives of the mother and the children, even after a divorce and the man's incarceration. Fights, distrust, and paralyzing fear were woven through all their interactions, including their conversations with their therapist, Marlene, one of my graduate students. As her clients related their history and current challenges, Marlene struggled under the weight of their despair. Watching her expressions and body language and listening to the tone of her voice, I half expected her to say, "Oh, you poor dears!" She didn't, at least not directly, but her pity was palpable.

After the session was over, I told her I sensed that she was feeling sorry for her clients and asked how she saw this affecting her therapeutic work. She said she considered compassion an essential piece of good therapy. I agreed, but said I thought it was important to distinguish between compassion and pity.

Compassion plunges us inside our clients' experiences, providing the means for fullbodied, empathic entry into their pain. It allows us to imaginatively feel ourselves as them. Pity, by contrast, is a toe-dipping enterprise. We feel *for* our clients, while we stay safe and distant, "professionally" removed. Pity reassures us that we are different from our clients.

I sensed that Marlene was keeping herself separate from the "unfortunate" people who sought her services and that this was hindering her ability to be helpful. I asked what would happen if she could see her clients as resourceful. How would her emotional response shift if she saw their wounds as signs of strength, if she appreciated their experiences as contributing to, rather than detracting from, their potential?

Marlene's sensitivity to her clients' pain provided her with half of what was necessary to work effectively. "You need to be able to recognize enough of your clients' misery to hold onto how horrible their plight is," I said. "But if this is all you do, your despair will hold you back and you'll only feel sorry for them."

Gregory Bateson wrote about the "bonus of understanding" made possible by double description. Recognizing that depth perception results from combining information from two different perspectives, Bateson proposed that "an extra dimension" of understanding results from bringing together two or more sources of information. With this idea in mind, I thought Marlene might benefit from practicing a kind of double *vision* or double *feeling*.

I suggested that each time someone in the family told Marlene something horrible about the past or present, she intone a transformative, two-word mantra to herself. The mantra would complement the pity she was already feeling, and the combination of the two points of view would make possible a new dimension to her felt-understanding. I stressed that the mantra was something to be intoned silently, privately—something to reconfigure her response to what she was hearing.

My use of the word "mantra" no doubt led Marlene to expect that the two words I was about to suggest would have serious spiritual overtones, evoking something formal or solemn. In fact, I had in mind more the playful, bright-eyed-wonder side of spirituality, but she didn't know that, so I think she was surprised by what I proposed.

"Okay, so here's the mantra: 'Oh, cool!' "

"Oh, cool?" she asked, a little incredulously.

"Yup. If you can respond to each of their stories of tragedy with a silent 'Oh, cool!' you will have transported yourself into understanding that symptoms and horrible histories can be resources for change instead of reasons for pity. Rather than be afraid of their problems, you can become curious about them, curious about how you and they can use them to create change."

Marlene may have thought I was cracked, but she agreed to take the mantra with her into her session. The pained expression disappeared from her face and, with it, her distance. She engaged, compassionately.

## Use Your Negative Reactions as a Transportation Device

Marlene moved from outside to inside the family, but she didn't get there by trying *not* to feel pity. When she attuned herself to the potential in her clients' pain, the pity took care of itself. Recognizing how such transformations work has helped me become a better supervisor. Now when my practicum students recoil from clients, I don't chastise them. Instead, I encourage them to use any negative reaction to their clients as a way of transporting themselves into their world.

Freed from having to strive for political correctness, my students don't have to try *not* to feel the way they do, and their reaction can become useful information, not only about them, but also, possibly, about their clients' friends and family. "If you," I say, "are feeling this way about your clients, maybe others are, too." Rather than trying to *take away* their feeling, I suggest they *complement* it with curiosity—curiosity about themselves (What's going on with me?), as well as about the clients (So what is it about these people, anyway? What don't I yet see? What don't I know?).

Such double feeling—estrangement balanced with curiosity—allows you to stay connected with yourself *and* transport yourself across any self-Other boundary you have imposed. Once you reach across into your clients' world, your recoiling will usually uncoil itself—at least it will when your reaching across reflects a genuine desire to know, rather than guarded reluctance to find out.

An overwhelmed single mother brought her twelve-year-old daughter to our clinic, wanting my team to "do something about" the girl's "bad attitude" and "nasty mouth." But the primary therapist and team members had trouble finding sufficient evidence of such behaviors. Charmed by the daughter's maturity and poise, and upset by the mother's dismissive tone and unrelenting negativity, they decided that the wrong person was being fingered as the problem. Partway through the second session, one of the therapists behind the mirror lost his patience with the mother and growled, "I just want to slap her!"

I whirled around in my seat, looked him in the eye, and said, "Excellent! Now take all the force of your frustration and disgust and use it to transport yourself into mother. Now! Go! Get inside her anger, far enough inside to feel the desire to slap your daughter! Slap that little smirk right off her face. And now keep listening to the session. Keep listening until you can grasp the daughter's desire to slap her mother or run away from home. As soon as you're there inside the daughter's experience, zoom back to the mother. And then back to the daughter. Back and forth and back again. When you can hold both desires simultaneously, you will be inside the *relationship*, and *your* desire to slap the mother will have probably disappeared."

## Lean Forward

I once invited a friend visiting from Germany, Jürgen Hargens, to talk for a few hours in a doctoral seminar I was teaching. Jürgen, a therapist and, at the time, the editor of a European journal on systemic therapy, came to class that day to discuss his constructivist approach to clinical work. One of the men in the class asked him many questions. If you were to read a transcript of the conversation, and if there were no indication of the student's tone of voice or nonverbal behavior, you might very well comment on his obvious fascination. But fascination has to do with leaning forward and asking, "What *is* that?" Instead, the student was leaning back, asking, "What is *that?*" The two phrasings define radically different relationships between a person and what he or she doesn't yet know. The first way of posing the question suggests, "Help me understand this from your perspective"; the latter, "I don't get what you're saying—but go ahead and talk about it some more; I'm happy to allow you to fail at convincing me to give a damn."

Encountering clients you consider to be Other, you need to find a way to become warmly fascinated. Otherwise, your conversation will sound painfully similar to my student's dialogue with Jürgen. You can certainly treat clients the way my son, Eric, critically examines and dissects foods he deems "exotic" (for many years, anything falling outside the four food groups—flour, cheese, ketchup, and chocolate), but the chances of your getting beyond a tentative and wincing exploration are slight. Far better to adopt something of the fascination of children in their second year of life. When Eric and Jenna were each first grasping the magic of language and the marvels of their surroundings, they were perpetual wonderment machines. Nothing was too scary or too yucky to stare at, taste, or use as lotion. From the moment they opened their eyes in the morning, they'd be reaching out to everything novel, demanding to know, "Wadaaaat?!" (Eric), "Badaaaah?!" (Jenna).[4] Of course, you can only orient this way to the new and different when you feel safe and comfortable.

## Recognize the Necessity of Feeling Safe

One of my students came to me one time for some advice about a male client she was seeing in her private practice. In his forties and still living with his parents, he wanted help in stopping his excessive and sometimes public masturbation. After the first couple of appointments, he had started masturbating in the session, and the therapist felt stymied. She didn't want to "become his mother" by telling him to stop, but she found it impossible to ignore his behavior. I talked with her about the necessity of her being able to relax during their conversations. As I saw it, she had three choices: seize on his in-session masturbating as an opportunity to explore the meanings (for him) of public masturbation and to experiment with ways of changing it; tell him she was willing to talk about, but not witness, his masturbation; or refer the case to someone else. The therapist was meeting with the man in an otherwise empty suite of offices on the weekend, so she didn't feel safe risking the first option, and she didn't want to give up on him. She chose to tell him that he couldn't masturbate in front of her, which established the necessary parameters for her to feel comfortable talking with him about changing his problem.

Physical safety is critical, but you also need to feel psychologically safe. I once took a case that otherwise would have been assigned to my supervisee, Irma. As I conducted the sessions, my team sat behind the mirror, observing. My decision to assume the role of primary therapist had resulted from a phone conversation I had had with the client, Mick, a burly Englishman in his midtwenties. A former crack addict who had remained clean for two years, Mick told me on the phone that he had recently started torturing his mother's cats when she was gone from the house. He had tried to stop his behavior on his own but had been woefully unsuccessful; all day at work he would feel a rush, a kind of high, he said, imagining what he would do to the cats when he got home. Anticipating Irma's reaction to this information, I told Mick that I worked with a team but that I would be his therapist. As it turned out, my decision was a good one. Irma is an animal activist, coordinating a spay and neuter program for homeless cats in Miami and working at the county level to create stiffer penalties for animal abusers. She was so horrified by what Mick told me in our sessions that she felt physically ill. She felt a modicum of relief when he told me at the beginning of the second session that he had killed one of the cats, for she knew that at least one of the animals was no longer suffering, but the news further confirmed for her that he was a monster, a sadist who deserved the same torture to which he had subjected the cats.

Gradually, over the next several weeks, Mick stopped, as he put it, "playing rugby" with the cats and, for the first time, began actively participating in the Narcotics Anonymous meetings he had been attending since getting off crack. The itch to hurt the animals waned, and he started talking about going back to school. After our fifth or sixth session, I asked Irma if she could now be his therapist. "Yes," she said, "because today he said he didn't feel the urge to go after the cats. But if the urge were to come back, I don't think I could."

The challenge is to be able to look for and find your clients' humanity while they are still strangers, *before* they do you the favor of making choices or taking action you consider acceptable. If, looking at a client, you see only a hopeless Other, therapy is out of the question. Before you can hope to be helpful, you need to be able to acknowledge (to yourself) your disgust, outrage, fear (or whatever) *and,* practicing double vision, become curious about the possibilities for change. You can't manage such a balance if you are achieving psychological (or, indeed, physical) safety by staying an outsider.

A therapist living in South America, Lucia, asked for a consult on her work with a young woman named Yaime. A few months before her first appointment, Yaime had broken off a marriage engagement, and the man had responded to her decision by brutally raping her. Fearing for her reputation in the community and knowing that, were her brothers to find out about the incident they would kill the man, Yaime, prior to coming to see Lucia, had kept the rape a secret. This had left her feeling vulnerable and full of fear, particularly since the rapist had contacted her at least four times since the incident.

Some time after therapy had begun, a woman named Carina called and asked for Lucia, saying she had a letter to give to her. Recognizing the woman's voice as Yaime's, Lucia suggested she deliver the letter in person. When Carina (Yaime) arrived, Lucia invited her in and asked her questions about her identity. Carina's responses—no, she didn't know where she lived; no, she didn't know whether she had a driver's license; and so on—concerned Lucia enough that she was afraid for the woman to leave. When Carina made for the door, Lucia blocked her way, telling her she wasn't going anywhere. Carina pushed her aside with surprising strength and dashed for the fifth-story office window. Lucia grabbed her before she could jump, threw her on the couch, and demanded answers. The woman said that because Yaime had allowed her to be hurt, she, in turn, needed to hurt, to punish, Yaime.

Lucia eventually allowed Carina to leave, and when Yaime came for her next appointment, Lucia could tell that she had no knowledge of Carina or the scuffle in the office. Over the next several appointments, various personalities appeared, including one with the same name as the rapist. At one point, Carina again showed up at the office, wielding a knife and threatening to stab both Lucia and Yaime. Lucia was terrified, not knowing how best to protect herself and her client. Carina seemed not only physically stronger than Yaime, but also more savvy (save for not knowing where she lived). Somehow, Lucia was able to prevent any violence, but she remained shaken.

On a few occasions, Carina had attended social events with Yaime's friends, and when the friends had called her *Yaime,* she had condescendingly corrected them. Considering her crazy, Yaime's friends began withdrawing from her. Lucia talked to Yaime about the possibility of hospitalization, but Yaime told her she would sooner die.

I suggested to Lucia that she assume Carina wouldn't have shown up if Yaime didn't need her. Following from this assumption, it made sense for Lucia to request a meeting with Carina, during which she could explain her understanding about Carina's importance in Yaime's life, to explain and show her respect for Carina's strength, and to apologize for how she had previously treated her. Lucia could then ask Carina about whether it was safe for her not to know where she lived, and if the two of them agreed that it was risky, Lucia might offer the possibility of Carina approaching Yaime for the necessary information. If Carina persisted in blaming Yaime for what had happened, Lucia could ask to be introduced to whoever had the most enlightened feminist sensibilities, someone who could advocate for a different placement of the blame. Carina was strong, but was she strong enough to stand up to the cultural assumption that women are responsible for men's misdeeds?

Finally, I suggested that Carina be given the idea of going "undercover," allowing herself to be called by the pseudonym *Yaime* so that she could successfully fool people who were too stupid to know who she really was. This would allow her to be around to help Yaime if she needed it, without jeopardizing Yaime's friendships or risking commital to a hospital.

Lucia was concerned about initiating a meeting with Carina, as she didn't want to implicitly support Yaime's using dissociated personalities as a means of coping. I pointed out that dissociation was Yaime's only way at the moment of staying safe, so Lucia would be best off embracing it as a starting place. Given that Carina was in the picture, she might as well be courted as an ally; attempting to banish her would, I figured, only make matters worse.

Six months after our consultation meeting, Lucia e-mailed me about the case.

> When I met with you, I was afraid because Carina had threatened to kill Yaime and me. Upon returning from the States, I approached all Yaime's personalities as different experiences of herself. I now consider them our assistants; they make an extra effort to come and tell us stories that we would otherwise not know. This change in perspective moved me from being terrified to being grateful: I now look forward to the arrival of any new personality. . . .
>
> I used your suggestion and told Carina that she could trick Yaime's friends by convincing them that she was Yaime. I did the same with a personality who wanted to take her place within her family. Both personalities

subsequently disappeared. For the last two months, no personality has expressed a desire to kill Yaime. They come saying they have important information to share with me so I may help her more!

Lucia's fear of Carina was legitimate, but her attempts to physically and psychologically protect herself and Yaime—preventing Carina from leaving, demanding answers from her, not wanting to initiate an appointment with her—kept Carina (and Yaime) as Other and thus heightened the danger. The situation turned around when Lucia accepted the legitimacy and importance of Carina and the others, when she welcomed them in from outside.

## Make Yourself Comfortable

If you are to tease out the hope, the strength, the potential in your clients' experience, you need to keep polishing that mischievous, playful sparkle in your eyes. No such polishing is possible until you feel physically and psychologically safe, but you also need to feel comfortable. Here's the rub, though—your eyes will never sparkle as long as you're trying to pawn off the responsibility for your comfort onto your clients. You've got to find a way, in the midst of the chaos and drama in the therapy room, to make *yourself* comfortable.

One of my supervisees was nervous that the young man who had come to see her because of marital problems was on the verge of telling her a secret. Not knowing how she'd handle such information, she told him she was ill at ease hearing things he wasn't saying to his wife: "I am honored that you trust me, but if I were your wife, I would feel kind of strange that you were coming to talk to a female therapist instead of me. You don't have some big dark secret you're wanting to spill, do you?" Sensitive to the cues being offered, the man shut up. He protected my supervisee by not telling her what she was too uneasy to hear. As a result, she felt relieved, but he was left in the lurch, for the moment he accepted her request to take care of her, he lost himself a therapist.

Another supervisee once asked a client, an intense professional man who seemed irritated by her questions, to "please not be too impatient" with her. He immediately softened and became solicitous, which helped her feel less flustered. Tension in the room decreased, but at the expense of the client's taking on the task of looking after her. How could he possibly relax into the relationship and trust the competence of his therapist as long as he was having to protect her? He couldn't and he didn't: A second appointment was scheduled but not kept.

Therapists get unnerved for other reasons, too, such as when their clients start arguing. A man I was supervising, Andrew, told an arguing mother and son that he couldn't meet with them unless they were willing to follow his two rules for therapy sessions. "The first rule is that no one interrupts or talks over anyone else. When one of us is speaking, the others must sit quietly and wait until that person is finished. The second rule is that each person must actually listen to and respect what the person who is speaking is saying. You don't have to agree with it, but you *do* have to respect it." Oh, if it were only that easy. Designed to lower Andrew's discomfort with the volume and chaos in the room, his rules, I suppose, worked to a degree: As everyone started walking on eggshells, a certain orderliness prevailed. But as Andrew became more traffic cop (or school principal) than therapist, the clients became tight-lipped and withdrawn, and the possibility for synergy quickly disappeared.

When Andrew came back for a consultation break with the team, I asked him if he could find a different way to go after his comfort. Rather than requiring his clients to supply it, could he, I wondered, find it by engaging with the clients *in their style?* "Instead of making them follow your rules, what if you followed theirs? Interrupt them, talk over them, welcome their conversational interaction as part of who they are." To illustrate the idea, I told him about a session I once had with a single mother and her rambunctious four-year-old twin boys. While she sat and talked about how overwhelmed she was, I stood up and, for the duration of the session, became a living jungle gym. As the boys climbed up one side of me and down the other, I got a workout, they had a blast, and the mother and I were able to engage in a peaceful conversation. Neither of us had to tell the boys to sit down or to behave or to stop interrupting.

Andrew returned to the session, abandoned his rules, and rolled up his sleeves. As he elbowed his way into the mother and son's argumentative style, as he allowed the conversation to heat up, as he kicked his damn eggshells out of the way, his eyes started sparkling.

## Distinguish Professional
## from Personal Intimacy

A student approached me with a dilemma. She understood, she said, the necessity of connecting with clients, but she was afraid that if she became *too* connected, she might become sexually attracted to them. For her and her clients' protection, she wanted me to help her find the proper "professional distance" from which to work—close enough to be helpful but far enough away to avoid sexual entanglements.

I suggested she rethink her assumption that sexual involvement is the inevitable end of a "continuum of closeness." By challenging this characterization, she might find other options for connecting with clients. Instead of thinking of all relationships as lying along a single continuum, what if, I asked, she allowed herself to distinguish different *types* of closeness? Medical students, for example, have to sort out the professional intimacy of seeing and touching a disrobed patient from the personal intimacy of seeing and touching a disrobed partner. Good doctors manage to keep the distinction firmly in place without sacrificing their or their patient's humanity and without sexualizing their scrutiny and touch.

We therapists, I said, are more likely than physicians to touch the *lives,* rather than the *bodies,* of our clients, but the benefits of distinguishing professional from personal intimacy remain the same. Unmeasurable on a "continuum of closeness," the difference is better captured in terms of the *pattern* of the intimacy or of the *expectations* of the people involved. In personal relationships, intimacy quite rightly depends and thrives on the expectation (and realization) of *mutuality*—mutual vulnerability, mutual attraction and desire, mutual sharing of stories, troubles, hopes, and so on. But in *professional* relationships, intimacy depends and thrives on what Bateson (2000) called *complementarity*—that is, on the *absence* of mutuality.[5] Our clients can trust us to the extent they know that we will not be responding to their requests for help with similar requests of our own.

We talked about how we therapists lose our freedom of response if we start wanting or needing something, *anything* (save for our fee), *back* from our clients.[6] If you take such freedom seriously, if you recognize that you can't operate as a therapist without such freedom, then you don't get personally invested in whether your clients care about you. I suggested to my student that she wouldn't have to adopt a position as an "outsider," wouldn't have to think about keeping her clients at a safe "distance," as long as she held expectations for complementary, rather than mutual, intimacy. This would allow her and her clients to become professionally connected *and* personally separated.

## *When You and Your Clients Aren't Yet of One Mind*

Crossing the boundary from outsider to insider precludes your viewing clients as Other and accords them the respect necessary for you to work with them. No longer strangers, you and they can talk as if you belong in the same neighborhood or as part of the same culture. But if you are to understand the *logic* of their predicaments—appreciating the choices they have made, breathing in the desperation they feel, sensing the strengths and resources they have at their disposal—you need a closer understanding than that of a friendly neighbor. You must cross not only the *self-Other* boundary—from outside to inside their culture—but also the *self-other* boundary, from outside to inside their heads and hearts. Such traversing requires you to exercise your metaphoric imagination, to structure your curiosity in terms of the metaphor, "I am you." You learn about your clients not by analyzing and diagnosing them from outside, but by hallucinating yourself inside their lives and looking around to see what you can discover.

### Tickle Your Metaphoric Curiosity

Some therapists believe that for you to be helpful, you must have lived through and successfully negotiated the same hell as your clients. Thus, goes the reasoning, you need children of your own to help struggling parents, be in recovery to help an alcoholic or addict, have survived sexual abuse to help a victim, and so on. From such a perspective, you have to have "been there" if you are to be trusted to know what it takes to change.[7]

Metaphoric understanding offers a virtual-reality alternative to the necessity of matching life histories. More than simply a feeling of empathy, it is a way of *making sense* of your clients' predicaments. As my clients tell me their stories, I imagine myself taking on their individual identities, not unlike, I would guess, the way an actor attempts to transmutate into the character he or she is playing.[8] During our sessions, I transport myself into their narratives, imagining myself experiencing their world with their bodies, speaking with their voices, perceiving the impossibility of their situations within the architecture of their beliefs.

Talking with Mick, attempting to understand his cat-torturing experience, I sought to breathe in his desire to hurt the "bleedin' little buggers," to feel his adrenalin rush as he chased and grabbed them, to drink in his fear of his mother catching him, to put on his mantle of shame. Without an embodied sense of these and other details from his experience, I couldn't have worked with him. I would have found it too easy to hold onto my animal-loving sensibilities and dismiss him (as he feared I would) as (in his words) "daft." But by imagining the two of us as one, by getting inside his "scrimmages" with the cats, I couldn't—and didn't feel the need to—retreat to the seeming psychological safety of moral indignation. I got to the point with him, as I try to with all my clients, where his situation, his behavior, his experience made sense. "Of course," I could think to myself, exercising my metaphoric imagination, "of course I can't stop thinking about the cats while I'm at work. Of course I get cotton mouth as I'm driving home. Of course I chase them—the little buggers are scared of me, so I *have* to go after them. Rugby time, mates! Of course."

Are you wondering how you will keep such empathy-spun unanimity from swirling you into bottomless despair? Once you've dived into the lived experience of your clients, what's to keep you from drowning? I hinted at a way earlier when I told you the story of my student, Marlene, using an "Oh, cool!" mantra to help her recognize the transformative possibilities of problems and symptoms. Within the concordance between you and your clients, you need the freedom to respond in unanticipated ways, to not get entangled in their beliefs, requests, and demands. The metaphoric structure of your understanding—"I am you"—entails not only a connection to your clients, but also a connected separation from them.[9] This is the shape of relational freedom.

## Use *Your* Experiences
## as a Port of Entry into *Theirs*

If you choose to imaginatively immerse yourself in the experience of your clients, you may at some point come face to face with yourself, or at least with what you fear you might be or might become. A clients' problem may resonate too closely with one of your own, or you may begin to question whether you're capable of making the same mistakes as your client or falling prey to the same desires. If, in metaphorically connecting with a person, you lose him or her or yourself in the process, you may need to transfer the case or at least find a different way of relating to your struggle.

A therapist whose work I was supervising was seeing a client who reminded her of herself. The more the client talked about her fights with her mother, the more the therapist found herself reflecting on her own unsatisfactory relationship with *her* mother. The effort to keep focused on her client, rather than herself, was exhausting her.

Contrary to the therapist's expectations, I suggested she not work so hard at returning her attention to her client. Instead of struggling to pull herself out of her own experience, what if, I asked, she were to explore it more thoroughly? If she did so *in the service of her client,* searching for jealousies, betrayals, disappointments, and so on in her own life, such discoveries might help her better understand her client's dilemma, and thus *effortlessly* transport her back into the therapeutic relationship. Once reconnected with her client, she could check out the accuracy of her self-informed understanding. If such a process enhanced and nuanced her appreciation of her client's experience, her personal life would no longer be getting in the way of her therapy; alternatively, if the process didn't result in a more accurate picture of the client's struggles, the therapist could be reassured that she was, indeed, *not* her client.

## Contribute Your Voice
## to a Two-part Invention[10]

Sitting behind the mirror one night in practicum, listening to a woman relay a series of painful details about her life, I was struck by the therapist's silence. When, after about forty minutes, he took a consultation break, I asked him why he had limited himself to the occasional head nod. He told me he wanted to show his respect to his client, "giving her the space to tell her story." I'm sure he felt respect for her, and, in the face of her overwhelming misery, he no doubt worried that whatever he offered would sound trite. But I disagreed with the idea that his client needed some kind of figurative "space" within which to talk.

If you conceive of therapy as place for people "to get stuff off their chests" (or, as you're more likely to put it when you're feeling less generous, "to dump"), then you're probably used to sitting still, listening quietly (or as I'm more likely to put it when *I'm* feeling less generous, "sitting numbly, listening dumbly"). Such a process inscribes a structural gap between you, rendering you an outsider: They go on and on and on, while you—bored, overwhelmed, irritated, whatever—glaze over.

But if you rethink therapy and your role in it, if you approach the process as an opportunity to *collaborate,* then your piece of the action changes. Rather than giving your clients the "space" for an uninterrupted soliloquy, you'll be looking for ways you can *participate* in their telling of their story, ways to lend your voice to a two-part invention. If, as I'm suggesting throughout the book, you're best off striving to become of one mind with your clients, you might as well start immediately, developing and *communicating* your metaphoric understanding of your clients' dilemmas.

## Communicate Your Metaphoric Understanding

Metaphoric understanding is essential if you are to find concordance with your clients. But, in and of itself, this isn't enough. Your clients need proof of your understanding; they need to know and trust that your grasp of their experience is accurate and in sync with theirs. You thus must do more than simply tell them *that* you understand— "Right, I know what you're up against"—you need to tell them, through your questions and empathic comments, exactly *what* you understand.

Jenna had a difficult time with teething, particularly when she was about eighteen months old. Waking up two or three times a night, she often had trouble going back to sleep. Shelley would nurse her for a while, and then I would walk her around until she drifted off. Her return to sleep was always provisional, though. If I jostled her too much while laying her down in her crib, or if Eric was thrashing around on his bed too loudly, all bets were off. Once again she'd be wide awake and I could count on at least another ten or fifteen minutes of walking before she would drift off again.

One night about 2 a.m., with Jenna relaxed and drowsy from nursing, her head resting on my right shoulder, I made my way down the

dark hallway to her room. Half asleep myself, I didn't notice her partially closed door until my left shoulder whacked into it, banging it
open and startling us both awake. "Oh no!" I winced to myself, "You
oaf! How could you?!!" I would have sunk into a pit of exhausted, reproachful frustration had it not been for a single empathic word spoken
softly in my right ear: "Ouch," Jenna said, melting my frazzled dismay.

Was this really an instance of toddler empathy? Jenna knew that
when you bump into something, it hurts, and when something
hurts, you say "ouch." My hearing her comment as an instance of empathy may have been overly generous, but child-development experts
would certainly support the notion that she, at that age, was capable
of empathic understanding. Regardless, her "ouch" diffused the
boundary separating a sleep-deprived father from his sleep-stealing
daughter. All of a sudden we were one, sharing the mutual plight of
my having further contributed to her inability to doze off.

By *demonstrating* your empathic understanding, rather than just
*claiming* you possess it, you give your clients the opportunity to trust
you, for they can hear when you're on the mark and can correct you
when you're off. As you, in trial-and-error fashion, adapt and fine-
tune your reflections, clients can better recognize themselves in what
you say. The more accurate you are in capturing their understanding
of their predicament, the more they will consider themselves and you
as being of one mind. Achieving such accuracy involves your reflecting back not only the content of their experience, but also something
of its emotional intensity and quality.

Many years ago I taught a course to undergraduates on "interpersonal communication." The students tended to want to sit quietly
and take notes, but this clashed with the content of the course and
my ideas about learning, so I looked for ways to infuse our conversations with drama. One day, I was attempting to get across the idea
that empathy is different from sympathy and that empathic communication involves more than just calmly and warmly repeating what
people tell you. I wanted them to grasp the idea that even yelling
could be experienced as empathic if it matches the passion and nature
of what the other person is thinking, feeling, and doing. To enliven
the idea, I invited one of the students, a football player named Jim
who outweighed me by eighty or a hundred pounds, to role play
with me.

"First," I said, "I will show you the *absence* of empathy." I placed two desks at the front of the class, ninety degrees to one another, and Jim and I sat down in them. I explained that Jim was driving a gleaming new sports car, a birthday present his folks had surprised him with just a week earlier. I was driving a dirty, rusted pickup truck, and I was about to run a red light. I hoped that Jim had his seat belt on because the crash was going to be pretty nasty. "Oh, by the way," I added, "your temper is pretty nasty, too. Really nasty." I then rammed his desk with mine, jumped out of my truck, surveyed the damage to his car, and yelled, "You idiot, look what you did!"

Jim was a quick study. He lumbered out of his car, took in a deep breath, and bellowed: "Look what *I* did?! What are you talking about?! You just ran a red and rammed into me! You totaled my car!"

"Okay kid," I sneered, walking toward him, "you can try that one on Daddy if he's stupid enough to believe you, but my headlight is busted and someone is going to pay for it!" I augmented my verbal attack with a shove, Jim responded in kind, and somehow in the next few seconds my shirt ripped open.

With the class (and me) a little in shock and before Jim's imaginary temper could cool down, we jumped back into our vehicles to do an instant replay. Again I ran a red, and again the sports car crumpled. Flinging open the door of my truck, I stomped over to Jim, yelling, "I bet you think I'm an idiot!"

"You *are* an idiot! You just ruined my car!"

"Here I am driving a worthless old truck and there isn't a scratch on it! And your brand-new car is totaled!"

"Right! Totaled!! What the hell were you doing? You ran a red light!!"

"You probably want to beat me to a pulp!"

"Absolutely!"

"Absolutely furious!"

"You got it!"

"So pissed, you haven't even noticed that cut over your eye. You hit that windshield damn hard! It must hurt like hell."

"Look at my car!"

"Just look at it! And look at you!" and then more softly, "What are we going to do about this mess? Are you okay?"

"Yeah."

At this point I stopped the role play and asked Jim if I, as the truck driver, was in any danger of being hit or of having my clothes further altered. Jim said that in some strange way he no longer felt angry with me—we were on the same side. I had managed to get inside his predicament, even though I was the cause of it. Empathy isn't about being nice.[11] I hadn't smiled once. Jim and I had yelled together, surveyed the damage together, fumed together about what an idiot driver I was. I found a way to move from outside to inside, knowing that even a football player won't rip the clothes of someone who isn't Other.[12]

My involvement in the second role-play differed significantly in one important respect from what I do as a therapist. By vociferously articulating Jim's position, I connected with him, but I did so as a manipulative means of protecting myself from him. The moment we were in sync on what he was thinking and how he was feeling, he no longer retained his emotional distance from me—in a sense, I robbed him of his anger by making it difficult for him to continue marking me as an outsider. In contrast, when I empathize with clients, I'm not attempting to *prevent* them from thinking or feeling anything, nor am I doing it for the benefit of *my* comfort or safety.[13] I empathize so I can appreciate and understand their predicaments as an insider and create the necessary rapport for therapeutic change. Let me give you an example from a therapy session—my first meeting with Mick, the guy who tortured cats.

Prior to the snippet of conversation below, Mick and I had been talking about what he had been doing to the cats, why he had sought help, and how he happened to be living in the States. He told me that his mother, who was partially aware of the "feline rugby matches," had threatened to throw him out if he didn't get help. He was holding down a job, but he didn't make enough to pay his own rent, so, for the last two years, he had been paying her a modest sum to live in an efficiency suite at one end of her house.

Born in the States, Mick grew up in England. When he was thirteen, his parents divorced and his mother moved to Miami; when he was sixteen, his father threw him out of their flat, and he took to the streets of London, getting involved with drugs and petty crime. Shortly after his twentieth birthday, he decided to pay his mother "an extended unannounced visit." She was reasonably pleased to see him, but soon they had "a falling out." For the next two years, Mick recreated his London lifestyle in Miami, and eventually the crack did him in. Desperate, he went back to his mother to ask for help in getting into a rehab center. She agreed.

MICK: I'll never forget the feeling when I went into that place [a detox unit]. The people. I mean, they're doin' just like me, but I felt like I didn't belong, God, not *me* in a Yank tank [American rehab]. [I thought] I wasn't that bad, not like these bleedin' Yanks, but I really was.

DOUGLAS: Can you describe it? As you walked through the doors and saw the others there?

M: It was just feeling ashamed at what I did, where I'm at, where I ended up. I used to despise those people and now I was no better. People were a little worse, people were a little better than me.

D: A really humbling experience.

I offered *humbling* as a summary of his description. He didn't tell me directly that I was off the mark; instead, he offered a different word.

M: It was a scary experience. . . . But going through this whole thing, I never wanted to kill myself over it. Because I always knew there was hope. That one day I'd get through it.

D: How did you know that?

I wanted to know how he knew there was reason for hope, in case I had occasion to use the information later on.

M: Just felt it.

D: Where?

I'm always curious about the location of an embodied understanding—the more specificity, the better.

M: In my gut I felt as long as someone would help me, I'd be all right. But I never had the guts to go up to someone and say, look, I do drugs, I'm all screwed up, I some need help. I never did that. I had nothing.

D: Except the feeling in your gut—that's all you had.

M: It was over. I knew it was over. It was all gone. The getting stoned—I couldn't get bulloxed [high] anymore. When I'd done drugs back home, I used to get the good high. Now that I've done it so much, I can't get that high.

D: Right.

M: I'm chasing that high that I can never get it. Never again.

D: Yeah.

My *right* and *yeah* may have given Mick the impression that I was with him, but I hadn't yet offered him (in this portion of our conversation) much reason to believe it.

M: It's like, going from doing a little piece, a five spot [roughly equilavent to what users in the States would call "a dime"], to doing a thirty spot [equivalent to "a fifty piece"] just to get stoned and that's not even getting me high. At one time.

D: Always just beyond your grasp.

M: Right. Yeah. . . .

*His* saying *right* and *yeah* confirmed that my statement accurately portrayed his experience.

D: So it sounds like there were two things going on in your gut. There was the feeling like "It's all over, there's nothing left," and the feeling, "I know that there's hope." Were there two [feelings], or were they the same thing?

I wanted to understand, as specifically as possible, how he made sense of his hope.

M: Basically the same. Basically the same. Two different feelings but basically the same. But I try not to look back at what I did. Right now what's going on with me now is what's bothering me more.

D: Hmm hmm.

M: You know it's like, my Mum says that the obsession has been lifted. I no longer have what you Yanks call the monkey on my shoulder.

D: Yeah.

M: That urge, that taste embedded in your head to where you can't get it out, and that's all you think about—it's no longer there. You know, I can now think a little clearer.

D: How long did it take you to get rid of it?

M: A year.

D: So you've had basically a free year here, where you felt free of the monkey.

He had already told me that he'd been out of rehab for "the better part" of two years, so I was just restating what he already knew I knew, but by *demonstrating* that I'd been listening, I gave him an opportunity to agree with me, agree that he'd experienced a kind of freedom.

M: Yeah. But then it was coming to where I had to deal with life.

D: Yeah.

M: And I'd get mad 'cause things don't go my way and I had to realize that things aren't always going to go my way. I gotta work for what I want. Don't steal it.

D: 'Cause you used to didn't have to think that way, right? If you wanted something, you'd go and steal it.

M: Steal it.

I offered my take on how things used to be, based on what he had just told me about the present. I didn't say anything new, but my comments extended the implications of his statement. I did the same thing with my next comment, and his response suggested to me that he accepted my interpretation.

D: And if things didn't go your way you'd get stoned and you wouldn't have to worry about it.

M: And I became good at what I did. I was real good at what I did. The stealing. The making people feel sorry for me so I could get my score. I'd sit somewhere and be humiliated just to get my score. To get my money. . . . I'd go to somebody and give 'em a sad story and cry and this and that. "Oh, I have no kip [no place to sleep], I have no dosh [money]." And in the end, I'd get what I want. I'd be

looking at them, shaking their hand, stealing their dosh, turn
around and laughing. And I had no fear of walking in somebody's
front door and walking back out with everything they had. And I've
done it.

D: So you were good at both manipulating people and also

M: Stealing, yeah.

D: Ripping them off.

M: Right.

I introduced *manipulating* as a summary of what he had told me,
and then, for no good reason, substituted *ripping off* for *stealing*. He
accepted the word switch, but if I could rewind the conversation and
try again, I would stick with his *stealing*: The more our word choices
match those of our clients and the more the clients agree with our descriptions of their experience, the fewer the differences between us
and, thus, the more concordance.

D: Did you rip off people you knew or people you didn't?

M: Anybody. Anybody I could get my hands on. I'm not proud of
what I did. I did what I had to do.

D: Are you proud of what you've *done?* In terms of

M: Getting better?

D: Yeah.

I used his statement about feeling *not proud* as an opportunity to ask
about his sense of accomplishment at getting off crack. Had we not
been in accord, he might have interpreted my question—"Are you
proud of what you've *done?*—as a sarcastic reference to his hurting the
cats; but he obviously knew what I was getting at, since he finished
the sentence for me. When I asked about his feeling proud, he mentioned his desire to make something of his life.

M: Yeah, I want to go to the Tech [to a training school], I want to do
things.

Once you know how to communicate your metaphoric understanding of your clients' dilemmas, you can *participate* in your clients'
storytelling, helping to ensure that you get the information you need
to be resourceful.

## Use Empathic Statements and Questions
## to Establish Pivot Points

Ever had clients who talked so quickly and with such focus and intensity that you couldn't get a word in edgewise? Watching from behind the mirror, I've seen many therapists twitch and fume as their attempts to stem the flow of their clients' stories, venting, or arguments have gone unheeded.

But how do you suppose the clients feel? If you were worked up about something and felt the need to get it off your chest, or if you were embroiled in an argument with that lame-brain spouse or no-good kid of yours, wouldn't you, too, ignore the insipid comments and questions of a nice little therapist who was politely trying to shut you up? But then if you continued to succeed in keeping the therapist at bay, you'd probably also feel like you'd wasted your money. Why bother coming back to see someone whose mouth hardly opened?

Rather than attempting to interrupt my clients, I work at connecting with them. As they tell me their story or demonstrate (with one or more other members of the family) their arguing style, I use empathic statements and questions to punctuate their narrative or interaction. By doing so, I help them know that I've got a handle on their experience, but I'm also able to create *pivot points*—opportunities for me to change the direction of the conversation or to get the perspective of someone else in the room. My clients don't feel shut down and I don't feel shut out.

Ester was fed up with the temper outbursts of her eleven-year-old son, Gordie, so she called our clinic, hoping to find someone who could "straighten him out." She told her therapist, a young woman on my practicum team, that despite being divorced for six years and dating the same man for the last three, she continued to be the victim of Gordie's temper, which would flare at any intimation of intimacy between her and her boyfriend.

A few weeks before our team saw Ester and Gordie for the third time, Ester's mother suffered a medical emergency. The family, along with Ester's boyfriend, had joined her in a nearby hospital's intensive care unit, supporting her and awaiting news about her condition. While they were sitting around, Ester noticed that her boyfriend had a thread hanging from the sleeve of his shirt, and when she went to bite it off, Gordie erupted. Ester had told us about it during the session following the hospital incident, but something inspired her to once again describe what had happened in this session a few weeks later.

ESTER: Last month, . . . [my mother was] lying in intensive care and my boyfriend had this string on his shirt.

GORDIE: Oh, my God.

E: And I went to remove it, but it wouldn't, it snagged. So my boyfriend said, "Bite it off." So I went to bite it off and he [Gordie] almost had a conniption. To the point where my father almost took off his belt.

THERAPIST: Right. You told me.

E: In the middle of the hospital! Screaming and ranting and "Ahhh!" and this and that because I went to bite a string off my boyfriend's shirt!

T: Okay.

E: That's not acceptable!

T: Right.

E: He has no *right* to do something like that! For *any* reason whatsoever!

The more Ester described the incident, the more upset she became, taking little if any notice of anything the therapist said. Up to this point, Gordie had stayed relatively calm, but when his mother provoked him with the following comment, he blew up.

E: I mean, my boyfriend wasn't lying on top of me, and even if he was—

G: [starts screaming profanities]

E: What is your problem?!

G: [continues screaming]

Overwhelmed, the therapist decided to take a break to consult with the team about how to get the session back on track, but Ester decided *she* was the one who needed to leave. Seeing the session going nowhere, she was ready to call it quits. The problem, from her perspective, was Gordie's.

T: I want to take a quick break.

E: *I'm* gonna take a break. I want to leave.

G: No!! Look at—

E: [dismissively] I want to leave. You talk to Gordie. I want to go outside.

Our clinic has phones connecting all the observation and therapy rooms, allowing supervisors to call the therapists with suggestions. I called in at this point, and the therapist tried to get Ester and Gordie to stop while she answered the phone.

T: Wait a minute. Hold on.

E: And I'm not going to do this anymore. I'm tired of this!

G: You always do this! You always do it!

Concerned that Ester would leave and not return, I offered the therapist over the phone the option of my coming into the room for a while rather than her coming back for a consultation. She agreed.

T: Hey. Um, can you stay here for a second because my supervisor

G: [continues screaming at his mother]

E: I'm just tired of this! I don't want to deal with this anymore! Look at this! Most women in the 90s—hello!—they meet a man, they start living with him. I've lived by myself. I have no friends because nobody will put up with him!

T: Right.

E: Okay. My life has become totally isolated, okay? The only one [her boyfriend] that's stuck around for three years is very, very good to me, and this is the way he [Gordie] reacts! I'm tired of it! I don't want to deal with this anymore!

I entered the room at this point and asked Ester if she would agree to sit down and talk for a bit. She reluctantly agreed. I began by acknowledging her and Gordie's frustration, pain, and desire to give up.

DOUGLAS: You know, it's clear for me from behind the mirror that obviously this is a very charged issue. No wonder you'd want to leave and no wonder that it brings tears. And I thought maybe we could use this moment to see whether we could get to a different

place with it. So if you're okay with kind of hanging around for a
minute, are you okay? With us talking?

E: There's a, what's your name?

D: Douglas.

E: Doug, there is no dealing with him! There's no reasoning! Delirious
in ICU and we're right in the room and he's, [starts to cry] there's
no excuse for that!

I began offering her my metaphoric understanding of her frustrated
helplessness and furious hopelessness.

D: There's no excuse and there's no reasoning.

E: No!

D: Nothing that you'd be able to say would make a difference.

E: No, nothing that you *can* say.

D: And you feel like you're being *imprisoned* by it, because you can't—

E: *All* the time, all the time. I don't have, I don't even have the ability
to say to my boyfriend one day, "Why don't you come over and have
dinner with us?"

My empathic statements shifted the interaction in the session from a
univocal tirade to a two-part invention. Listening and responding to
what I said, Ester quickly adjusted to the content *and* the pattern of
my interspersed comments: She began *expecting* me to sprinkle something into her telling of her story. I figured at this point I could safely
venture a question.

D: Do you notice, did you notice

E: No.

D: that when this happened, was it, was it a gradual buildup or was it,
like Gordie was saying, that it was an immediate thing?

E: It was immediate! Because he was standing here, I'm sitting in one
of those recliners, and my boyfriend was standing here, and I see
this string hanging off of his sleeve. I mean, he wasn't even sitting
on the, the, the hand rest of the chair.

Ester's description was *in response to my question,* so I was now able to
decide when she had given me sufficient information.

D: Right. Thank you.

Having connected with Ester through the empathic comments I had interspersed during her storytelling, I could now use any of my moments of "air time" to create a pivot point—to, in this case, turn to her son—without risking the loss of our unanimity. I wanted to give Gordie an opportunity to provide a reflective, rather than reactive, response to what his mother had described happening in the hospital.

D: Now. [turning to Gordie] When that happened, when you said you snapped into that—or your mother's term—can you describe what went on in your body when you saw that [his mother biting the thread]? What . . . did you experience when you saw that?

G: I don't know. [inaudible] I just, I felt like hitting something. It felt like,

D: Just automatic.

G: I felt like breaking something.

D: Right.

G: It was just like a rush, a complete rush.

E: [to Gordie] Any feelings for anybody in there at all!?

Had I let Ester, as angry as she still was, begin grilling Gordie about his lack of sensitivity, he, and the session as a whole, could have exploded in my face. Protecting my therapeutic freedom, I stopped Ester and further explored Gordie's experience.

D: [to Ester] Hang on, hang on. [to Gordie] So, in the middle, you saw it and all of a sudden, without ever even thinking, it was just automatic.

G: I didn't think about it, it just, it happens a lot, like a couple times before like, there's

D: Yeah.

Continuing to use empathic statements and questions to create pivot points, I went back and forth between mother and son, weaving their contributions together. During our three-way conversation (a *three-part invention?*), we established that Gordie had blown up in a variety of circumstances, whenever he felt humiliated or threatened. We also determined that his degree of upset was inversely related to how confident and strong he was feeling at the time. By the end of the session, Ester was exploring alternatives to yelling at and issuing threats to someone who was already feeling threatened, and Gordie was planning to draw pictures of martial artists who were able to defend themselves without needing to resort to violence.

## Adjust to Your Clients' Rate
## of Thinking and Talking

In the hypnosis class I teach, I typically give the students a series of interpersonal assignments. One week they are to go out into the community and find someone who talks more slowly than they do. Engaging the person in conversation, they are to slow down to his or her rate of speech and notice what happens. In subsequent weeks, I ask them to make analogous matching adjustments with people who speak more quickly, more softly, and more loudly. Most students find the exercises challenging but invigorating. The interpersonal stretching convinces at least some of them that they are more adaptable than they would have predicted.

One of my practicum students, Murray, had taken the class, but the exercises hadn't helped him alter his conversational mannerisms. Very frequently—and, as far as I could tell, randomly—he would murmur "okay" or "uhh huh" as he listened to his clients talking. He did the same thing when chatting with me, so I was able to give him a firsthand account of how his ongoing sprinkling of these "little affirmations" affected me.

"Murray, I feel like slugging you," I explained. "I'm sure you're paying attention to what I'm saying, but if I didn't know you, I'd think you were trying to hurry me along, to not-so-subtly get me to finish up and shut up. Stop nudging your clients to speak more quickly. Your job is to adapt to *their* speed of thinking and talking, not to rev them up to *yours*." After watching some videotapes of his therapy sessions, Murray could identify what he was doing, and he was able to significantly reduce the number of, and to more appropriately place, his affirmations. When I congratulated him on his success in making the change, he joked that it would probably improve his marriage, given that his wife had often complained of his not listening.

I started giving the stretching assignments in my hypnosis class after watching therapists get out of sync with their clients' rate of responding to their comments and questions. One woman, a self-described "fast-talking New Yorker," would get impatient and anxious when the thoughtful, taciturn man with whom she was working failed to provide her with an immediate comeback to one of her questions. She'd follow up with a second question, and then a third and a fourth, and then she'd start supplying possible answers. He'd sit back, a little stunned, while she carried on both sides of the conversation: "What do you think it would take for you to try something new this week? Or are you ready to do something new? Maybe you need some more time, do you think? Or maybe we could look at defining a different goal. Or at least fine-tuning the one we came up with. Do you want to go slow for a while and see what happens? Then we could start next session seeing what if anything is different or needs to be different and then that would be a good time to figure out about the goal, whether it needs to be changed. Or not."

I called in and suggested she slllooooooowwwwwwww dooooowwwwwwwwnnnnn, and I passed along the advice of one my teachers, Monte Bobele: "Ask one question at a time. Get the answer to the first before going on to the second."

## Speak with the Strength of *Their* Convictions

If you're an upbeat person, or if you're unsettled by strongly expressed emotions, you might find yourself trying to attenuate the severity or seriousness of what your clients are saying. Do this, and you risk communicating to them that you're afraid of what they're saying, afraid to be of one mind with them. If a man tells you that everything is so hideous that he sometimes thinks a gun to the head would be the best solution, you aren't going to help him feel less desperate or hopeless by responding with a nicer, tidier version. Instead of responding, "You must be feeling kind of bad," hang out with him inside his despair: "Blowing your brains out sometimes seems like the only way out." Once you can resonate with your clients wherever they happen to *be*, and once they trust that you aren't going to nice-ify what they tell you, you and they together can use the resulting concordance as a stepping-stone to where they might *head:* "If, instead of your brains, you were to blow the *cobwebs* out of your head—you know, really do a thorough spring cleaning of your mind—what do you suppose you'd stumble across?"

## Offer Thanks to Anyone (or Anything) but Clients

The merchants in the outdoor bazaars in Turkey had my number. The moment I walked into a shop, the owner would send a young boy off to buy me a small glass of chai (tea). The drink probably cost the equivalent of a penny or two, but I felt somehow beholden when it was handed to me (or even before then—the feeling of obligation began creeping up on me as soon as the boy was dispatched). As the recipient, now, of a small kindness, I couldn't just up and leave. I felt it necessary to at least stay and finish the drink, if not to purchase something, *anything,* however inexpensive. I was aware of the business acumen behind the merchant's treating me as a guest, but I *still* felt indebted, still felt caught in the interpersonal web of his gift-giving.

Carl had the habit of warmly thanking his clients for coming to their appointments, and when I heard him do it one night in practicum near the beginning of the semester, I found myself sipping those twenty-five-year-old memories of Turkish chai. "It's one thing," I said to him, "if your clients want to schedule their next appointment because they're getting something out of coming, but it's quite another if it's because they somehow feel obligated. When you thank them, you let them know that you're grateful, that *you're* getting something from their coming. If they sense from the warmth of your gratitude that you somehow *need* them to come back, they may feel pulled to do so as a way of thanking you for the help you've provided them. You want to ensure that if they return for another appointment, they're doing it for *themselves,* not for you."

Carl thought over what I said, and when he came back to practicum the following week, he said that in keeping with my notions of not negating unwanted behaviors, he had decided to maintain his thanking but to change who (and what) he thanked. True to his word and the twinkle in his eye, he spent the rest of the semester warmly thanking me, his colleagues, the table behind the mirror, his Palm Pilot—everyone and everything who wasn't a client.

## Give Your Clients the Freedom
## to be Themselves

With all this talk about becoming of one mind with your clients, I guess I should clarify that you only do this in the service of allowing them to be themselves. Once their appointment is over, you go onto other clients, to new concordances, and they go home without you. They may take your suggestions along with them, but not your *embodied* presence.

A therapist I was supervising asked a couple she was seeing, "So, we had a good Father's Day?" Later in the session, she inquired, "So, we mentioned our concern to Jack [their son]?" If I had been her clients, I'd have felt as if she were trespassing, and I'd have wanted to set her straight: "It was *my* damn Father's Day and *my* damn conversation with my son. *You* weren't there!" With this in mind, I suggested that she alter how she phrased her questions, ensuring that she not elbow her way into her clients' experiences, choices, and actions. "How was your Father's Day?" "Did you mention your concern to Jack?"

## Invent *Intra*ventions

Once I can make insider sense of my clients' experience—their actions, thoughts, circumstances, and emotional reactions—I can begin to wonder about opportunities for change, about the possibilities embedded within their impossibilities.[14] If you start musing about change too soon, while you're still an outsider, you risk coming up with ideas that are nothing more than interventions (from the Latin, *inter,* between + *venire,* to come: to come between)—suggestions from outside, extraneous ideas, designed to *come between* your clients and their problems. I prefer, instead, to cast about for what I call *intra*ventions (from the Latin *intra,* on the inside, within + *venire,* to come)—suggestions from *inside* the concordance between my clients and me, ideas designed to alter (not negate) the relationship between the clients and their symptoms. Such an approach frees me from the demanding delusion that I as the therapist need to be "the creative one," the knowing expert who diagnoses pathologies and prescribes interventive solutions. When your clients trust your insider understanding, when they know you know, you and they are in a good position for inventing intraventions.

For example, when Joannie experienced her arm pain as poison, I intraventively suggested that given the presence of poison, an antidote must obviously be available (see the Introduction). The notion of applying an antidote to the pain made insider sense. And when the poison lingered, I intraventively defined it, and Joannie intraventively accepted it, as a homeopathic remedy.

You'll find another example in Chapter 2. Mac's adult children, you'll remember, asked me to use hypnosis to make him eat. Had I agreed to do so, my efforts would have taken the shape of an intervention, coming between Mac and his closed throat, attempting to force his body into compliance. Instead, Mac's and my *intra*vention helped to protect the integrity of his not eating and to preserve his identity as a strong man—strong enough, still, to stubbornly resist the efforts of his kids to make him follow their dictates.

Other illustrations of intraventions—suggested and accepted changes that fit within the pattern and logic of the clients' experience[15]—are sprinkled throughout the rest of the book.

## Learn from Antonio Banderas

Remember the scene in *The Mask of Zorro* where Anthony Hopkins (playing the aging Don Diego de la Vega) teaches Antonio Banderas (a young street thief) an important lesson in the art of sword fighting? Hopkins, looking distinctly unimpressed, watches as Banderas, full of bravado, pierces and slices the air with an impressive flurry of thrusts and parries. With no warning and minimal effort, Hopkins casually but swiftly brings his sword up and around, slapping away his protégé's weapon with a smooth, easy swipe.

Supervising from behind a one-way mirror, I've watched this same exchange played out countless times in the therapy room. Even without Hopkins's Welsh accent and blue eyes, many clients—particularly teenagers and other involuntary clients—can muster an impressive imitation of his teaching technique. Faced with an earnest therapist who's reaching out with unsolicited recommendations, they respond with an unceremonious "Hopkins's swipe."

The following conversation took place just after Kellie, a young teenager, had been complaining to her therapist, Carol, about not getting along with the girls in her classroom. Carol jumped into action, offering a succession of ideas about what Kellie could do to improve her situation. Each time Carol extended a suggestion, Kellie effortlessly knocked it out of her hand.

CAROL: Do you think it might be helpful to talk to your teacher about this?

KELLIE: No. I've tried all week. She just tells me to get in my group.

C: Sometimes its helpful to ask Mom or Dad to schedule a conference to talk to a teacher.

K: That wouldn't work—I need to do it myself.

C: Well, so, between this week and next, why don't you try to schedule an appointment with your teacher? Maybe after school.

K: I can't—I ride the bus.

C: How about during lunch?

K: I don't want to go during lunch because I like being with my friends.

Later in the session, Kellie talked about her difficulty adjusting to her parents' decision to divorce, and Carol once again reached forward in an effort to help.

C: There are some really good books about this. Do you like to read?

K: Not really.

Before committing yourself to any particular course of action, find out what your clients want from you, what they've already tried to do to solve their dilemma, and what they're good at, like to do, are willing to try, and so on. If you casually check this out while you're chatting, you'll avoid casting them as a smug Anthony Hopkins and you as an embarrassed Antonio Banderas.

### Structure Your Reframes Inductively

Sometimes, before clients can try doing something new in response to a situation or problem, they need first to change the way they're thinking about it. But shifting their perspective of their experience—or, as the MRI folks would say, "reframing" it[16]—can prove difficult. If you want to up the chances that your clients won't summarily dismiss your reframe, that they will risk shifting their beliefs or their understanding of their predicament, you'll do best to inductively structure your delivery of ideas.

With inductive reasoning, you move upward from the specific to the general, deriving an encompassing principle or idea from a set of particularities. When you offer a reframe inductively, you start by summarizing the details of your clients' situation as you understand them. One detail at a time, you confirm the specifics of what they've told you. Once you and your clients are in agreement—unanimous—about the particulars, you can then offer a new understanding of how the pieces fit together—a reframe that casts the pieces in a new light.

Kiri had been living with Matt for seven years when she came to see a therapist in our university clinic for help in understanding him. They had been married for a few years and were still living together, but Kiri had decided she wanted out of the marriage. Recently, after listening to some talk shows focusing on sexual issues, she had decided she needed to speak with an expert about some of her husband's sexual proclivities. She thought if she could get answers to her questions, she would understand better what had happened to them, and this would help her move on. The therapist suggested that she and Kiri meet with my wife, Shelley, who teaches and writes about sexuality. Unfortunately, Shelley wasn't able to accommodate their request, so she, in turn, referred them to me.

I began our two-hour consultation session by clarifying with Kiri how she had ended up seeing me rather than Shelley, explaining how Shelley and I are both faculty in the same department and that we co-teach, on occasion, a course on sexuality and sex therapy. Kiri asked how it was for each of us working with the other, "because that was my and my husband's biggest thing. We worked together for several years. He was my boss." The hardest thing was "seeing each other all the time, never having the opportunity to miss each other."

During the first few years of their relationship, while they were living together but before they married, Kiri and Matt had had "great sex," making love once or twice a week. But for a long time, they had been "like roommates," sharing no intimacy. Back when they were still working together, they usually drove to the office together, but after a while, he started, about once a week, suggesting she go on ahead, and he would show up an hour or two later. When she'd get home, she'd notice that he'd changed the sheets, and "apparently he had been relieving himself on them."[17] She told herself this was okay, as long as it wasn't affecting their sexual activity together.

Gradually, the frequency of Matt's arriving late at work increased and the frequency of their lovemaking decreased. Never having been the one to initiate sex, Kiri was reluctant to say anything, but one day she steeled herself and asked to be included in his masturbating: "I just want you to know," she told him, "I want you to come to me, I don't want you to think you can't come to me to relieve yourself. We can make it fun." She sensed, but wasn't sure, that he was shocked and a little embarrassed that she knew what he was doing with his Penthouse magazines. He thanked her for being supportive but never took her up on her offer.

Rebuffed and devastated, Kiri left him alone. Some months later, they decided to start a family; their sexual relationship improved while they were working at conceiving, but when Kiri became pregnant, Matt stopped touching her and wanted nothing to do with her sexually, despite her increased arousal. Attributing his sexual distance to his being distracted by the pressures of a new job and "being freakish" about her growing belly, she let him be, never confronting him. Instead, she looked forward to a time after the baby would arrive, hoping things would improve once her figure returned to normal. But Matt continued not being interested in sex after the baby was born, inspiring Kiri to speculate with her girlfriend that his witnessing the birth had probably negatively affected his ability to see her in a sexual way.

At the time of our appointment, Kiri's child was two years old, and she and Matt hadn't had sex for three years. I commented on how hard she had worked at coming up with plausible reasons for his lack of sexual interest in her, and I asked what had prevented her from checking out any of her speculations with him. She complained about how exhausting it was to be continually thinking up excuses for him, but regarded this as much less dangerous than sitting him down and demanding to know what was going on. Afraid that he would tell her he didn't find her sexually attractive, she had never once questioned him directly about his experience of their sexual (non)relationship or about his "relieving himself."

Assuming that her reluctance to confront Matt had to do with her shattered self-confidence, Kiri speculated that she would be able to talk with him about the issues a few years in the future, once the marriage had been formally terminated and they had had a chance to become friends again. In the meantime, she felt trapped and stifled, unable to move forward. She hoped I could supply the explanations that she was too insecure to demand from Matt, and that these explanations would give her the necessary shove to walk out of the marriage.

I didn't see much potential benefit in my giving Kiri a hearsay-based diagnosis of Matt's sexual behaviors, but I did think that if her experience could be reframed in some way, it might free her up to get the answers she wanted from the person who had them. A possible reframe came to mind right at the beginning of the session, when she mentioned the respective capacities in which she and Matt had worked together. But I kept it my back pocket for the next hour, while I gathered information and inductively laid the necessary foundation for offering it to her.

I can't show you an hour's worth of foundation laying, but I can illustrate and comment on some of what I was doing in the few minutes prior to introducing the reframe. At this point in the conversation, Kiri had just been telling me about Matt's using their home computer for internet-based sexual gratification.

KIRI: Apparently you can get a lot of things on the internet.

DOUGLAS: Not work related. Did you walk in and see him doing that?

K: No, I would never want to embarrass him, to walk in on him. But just listening to the sounds on the computer, I could tell he wasn't working. I heard pornographic sounds.

D: And you didn't confront him on it.

K: Instead I just became this angry person. Very distant.

D: Does he know that you know about the cybersex?

K: No. I know, a lot of this is me never approaching him on this.

D: You've said a couple of things about the not approaching, so let me check it out and see if you agree. You've been protecting him a lot over the course of the marriage. . . . You've not confronted him, didn't want to embarrass him, you've made excuses for him—"He's tired, he's working hard,

K: Hmm hmm.

D: "his job isn't going well, he's trying to figure out what he wants to do with his career, he's upset, he's perhaps not able to be attracted to a pregnant woman, perhaps he can't be attracted to a woman who's given birth."

These were all details that she had talked about earlier in the session.

K: Hmm hmm.
D: You've done a lot of anticipation,
K: Yes.
D: and protection of him.
K: Hmm hmm. Yeah, that's true. . . .

She agreed with my assessment. She'd never confronted him, and she'd worked hard to protect him.

D: So can you talk a little bit about, or is there more, about your not confronting or the not asking? Because you're obviously very curious, you've been curious for years.

I wanted to make sure I hadn't missed anything, and I wanted to understand how she made sense of it.

K: Yeah. I just, I guess in my mind, I'm thinking, "How could anybody prefer masturbation over—?" [laughs] I mean, I always thought men would just prefer that, even if the woman is, like, terribly unattractive. I mean they would just put a bag [laughs] over her head. I mean, emotionally, what could be going on?

She told me about her confusion, about what she wanted to know, but she didn't answer my question, so I asked it again.

D: So you *are* terribly curious?
K: Hmm hmm. . . .
D: So what is it about the curiosity that it hasn't carried you into saying, "Ah, Matt, I've got a question for you."
K: Because I'm scared. I'm a little embarrassed.
D: It makes you vulnerable.
K: Hmm hmm.
D: Because he might say something you don't want to hear.
K: Hmm hmm. . . . But . . . normally, I would be the type that even though I felt it at the moment, I wouldn't say it just because it

would hurt his feelings. Because I'm always, I find a pattern with myself, I'm always protecting him.

Kiri attributed her reluctance to fear and embarrassment. Somehow she just wasn't strong enough to ask him directly. But she also recognized that she was protective.

I'd now laid the necessary groundwork to offer my reframe, to suggest an understanding of why she was both fearful *and* protective. In this instance, I presented the idea in the form of a question.

D: Yeah. Have you ever stopped being his employee?
K: What do you mean?
D: He was your boss.
K: Hmm hmm.
D: It's very, very difficult to look your boss in the eye and say, "I'm holding you accountable." Bosses don't get confronted.
K: [quietly] I never even thought about it in that way. [long pause] Wow. [laughs, then a long pause] You might have something there. [laughs] I guess because I've always looked up to him.
D: Yeah.

After asking me to explain my question about whether she'd ever stopped being an employee, Kiri accepted my reframe with open arms. I suppose it's possible she would have done the same if I'd asked the question when I first thought of it, back at the very beginning of the session when she mentioned that her husband had been her boss, but if she hadn't, I would have been in the position of trying to *prove* to her that the reframe made sense. And if she had been at all reluctant to entertain the idea, I'd have had a long uphill battle ahead of me.

I don't want to try to convince people who have their arms crossed, who are nonverbally saying, "Prove to me that I should listen or believe what you're saying." You can avoid having to bolster or shore up a reframe by not presenting it until you and your clients know that you know the particularities of their situation. Offer your new way of perceiving their situation only after you and they are of one mind concerning the building blocks of your premise.

## Offer Reframing Rather than Reframes

Some therapists, influenced by the Milan team's early work (Selvini Palazzoli, Boscolo, Cecchin, & Prata, 1978), treat reframes as succinct, one-shot messages you deliver to your clients, soliloquies that you drop like bombs just before you end your sessions and bolt from the therapy room.[18] The Milan team would refuse to address their clients' confusion or respond to their questions, arguing that the impact of the message would be diminished by their continuing to talk about it.

Such an approach may be necessary if you aren't clear about the idea you're offering, or if you're afraid that if you talk too much about it with your clients, you'll mess up and let it dissolve into nonsense. But if you're confident about your reframe, why not help your clients try it on for size?

I think of a reframe as a pair of polarizing glasses, a perception-altering device that allows me and my clients to experiment with a new and more liberating way of making sense of their situation. Thinking *intra-* rather than *inter*-ventively, I want to make sure the glasses work (i.e., refract information) effectively, so I'll engage in conversation long after first introducing my context-altering idea. The reframe thus becomes a refram*ing*—an ongoing process of redefining.

Kiri and I continued to talk for almost an hour after I offered her my initial reframe. Again and again, I used the idea of her being a loyal employee to make sense of new information she shared, and I listened for the times when she herself used the idea to make sense of what had been happening.

K: We had a really good relationship before—before getting together.
D: It's very possible to have a good boss-employee relationship.
K: Hmm hmm.
D: And it's very possible to have a good relationship between equals.
K: Hmm hmm.
D: What's difficult is having a boss-employee relationship dressed up like a relationship between equals.
K: Hmm hmm. . . .
D: So there's a lot of employee loyalty.
K: Yeah.
D: And at the same time, you're also trying to find a way to have an equal voice.

K: Hmm hmm. [long pause] I think I should have done that a little bit earlier in the relationship.

D: It could be that had you done that earlier, the relationship would have ended then.

K: Hmm hmm. [long pause] I think it would have saved me a lot of— [laughs]

D: Well, I would imagine that if it were a marriage between equals, you would have said, "Hey Matt, whatcha doin'?"

K: Hmm hmm.

D: Certainly it's still vulnerable to ask someone a question that potentially means their saying, "I don't find you attractive."

I didn't want to discount what Kiri had already told me about her fear of being directly rejected by Matt, so I made sure to account for it within the reframe. I was still thinking inductively, using the details of what she'd described to support the orienting notion of her relating to her husband like a boss.

K: Hmm hmm.

D: But it's a lot easier to ask that question of someone who is your equal than somebody who's your boss.

K: Hmm hmm, hmm hmm.

D: Because bosses who get asked those sorts of questions fire the employee.

K: Hmm hmm. I think I've always set myself up that way. . . . Well, that tells something about me. [laughs] . . . So loyal, huh?

D: Yeah, extremely loyal. Loyalty's a marvelous thing, you know. It works also between equals, but it is different from loyalty to somebody who's your boss.

K: Hmm hmm.

D: Because the loyalty to a boss is such that you can never question. The loyalty to somebody who's your equal is that you're being loyal by *virtue* of questioning. In a sense, the loyalty of you as an employee has kept you silent—which is the proper thing to do in that position.

Near the end of our time together, I asked Kiri if she'd gotten from our session what she'd hoped for.

K: I'm still so bothered about the sexual issue. I think I'm ready to
just hear [from Matt] whatever it is. [laughs] I think it will give me
strength to say, "You know what?"

This was a significantly different position from where she had been a
few hours earlier. In response, I reinvoked and highlighted the reframe.

D: You'll be able to hear his answer, knowing you're not his employee
anymore, whether you say that directly to him or just say it to
yourself.
K: Hmm hmm.
D: But for you to be able to hear it from somebody who's not your boss
will put a very different spin on it than if you were hearing it from
somebody you revere and have loyalty toward and can't question.
K: Hmm hmm.
D: To be able to free yourself up to question and to be curious and to
want answers.
K: I think for me to take that step, to actually ask him,
D: Hmm hmm.
K: would be relinquishing this employee. I really do—because why I
haven't questioned this for five years. [laughs]

She was making sense of her experience within the reframe.

D: It makes good sense why you haven't questioned it for five years.
K: Hmm hmm.
D: You're not allowed to if you're an employee.

I should have waited for *her* to say this.

K: Hmm hmm.
D: But you've kept from getting fired.
K: Hmm hmm. I'm sitting here—can you believe this?—saying, "No,
wait until he's physically moved out and you are actually divorced
and *then* ask the question." Again, I'm like confirming that, "You
know what? Wait until either you quit or you're fired, and then you
get to question." But you know what? I should have the right to
question! [laughs]

D: As his wife you do. Sure.

K: That's the problem. I've never really put myself—

D: You've never really been his wife.

K: Put myself, it's always been, oh my God. Oh.

I offered a tangible way for her to handle that "oh my God" reaction, recommending a book that continued to underscore the reframe.

D: Ever seen the book, *What Color is Your Parachute?*

K: A book? Who is it by?

D: By a guy named Bolles. It's about what to do when you get fired or you quit and you're looking around for a new job.

K: Hmm hmm.

D: You might find it interesting, except—

K: Just apply it to my life.

D: Yeah. What you've found is, you've just quit. Congratulations. [I reach forward and shake her hand]

K: Thank you. [the therapist who had requested the consult shakes her hand, too] Wow. I never would have, I've always been, always been concerned about what he's thinking, or what he's feeling, or am I going to hurt his feelings or, God! It's the exact same feeling I had when I was *working* for him. [laughs, then a very long pause] Wow. Thank you.

The reframing provided Kiri with a parachute, allowing her to jump to freedom—the freedom to question and choose as an equal.

## Offer Ideas in Bite-sized Pieces

In the practicum sessions I supervise, the therapists usually take a consultation break partway through so that they, the team, and I can gather our thoughts, reflect on what we've learned, and construct an idea (sometimes a reframe) or a suggestion that we can then offer as a message to the clients. Many times I've seen good therapists take a good message and deliver it badly—as a nonstop, no-pause-for-a-breath soliloquy. More often than not when this happens, the clients leave confused.

Perhaps if you think of the idea you want to convey as a good meal (whether you conceive of yourself as a chef or a short-order cook), you'll find it easier to present it to your clients so as not to choke them.

Arrange the whole of it into bite-sized portions, and offer one piece at a time, making sure you give your clients time to digest the first one before offering the second, the second before offering the third, and so on.

How do you know when they're ready for the next piece of your idea? Watch their eyes. Typically, as they're sorting through what you've said, making sense of it, they'll look away from you. While their eyes are elsewhere and their focus is inward, shut up and wait. Once they renew eye contact, offer the next piece.

If you look back over the excerpts from my session with Kiri, you'll notice how many times she said "hmm hmm" to me. Part of that had to do with the way I portioned out my comments—I gave her one bite-sized piece at a time, and waited till she told me with her eyes and her "hmm hmm" that she was ready for me to continue. And when she needed more time to chew over what I'd said, I honored the silence.

## Assess Your Relationship with Clients

Whenever I get bogged down in therapy, I start asking myself questions about my relationship with my clients:

- Am I still an outsider? Why? What am I doing?
- Am I responding to them as Other?
- Do I feel safe transporting my imagination into their lives, reaching for a metaphoric understanding of their experience? Am I comfortable?
- What have I failed to notice or appreciate? Is my double vision allowing me to see pain *and* possibilities?
- Am I *communicating* my metaphoric understanding in a way they can trust?
- Am I offering them *intra-* rather *inter*-ventive suggestions?
- Am I presenting my ideas and reframes in digestible portions?

If my clients and I are not yet of one mind, I want to make sure that my assumptions, attitudes, emotional responses, ways of thinking, and ways of communicating aren't getting in the way. Once I'm able to think, feel, and speak like an insider, I can then attend therapeutically to how my clients are relating to me and what I have to offer, as well as how they're relating to themselves. These are the subjects of the next two chapters.

# 4

# Your Clients' Relationship with You

A boy . . . arrived [at Summerhill School] so full of pent-up aggression after years of being bullied and labeled an academic failure at a smart private school that he threw stones through twenty-two windows. When he was aiming for the twenty-third, [A. S.] Neill [the founder and headmaster of Summerhill] appeared beside him, picked up a stone, threw and missed. The boy laughed and never broke another window. Instead he calmed down, made friends and spent two terms playing solidly before going to lessons.

*—Angela Neustatter*

In Chapter 3, I talked about the necessity of getting inside the world—the culture, the head, the heart—of your clients. But if you are to be helpful, they also need to step into *your* world, to enter a relationship ostensibly devoted to therapeutic change. Taking such a step can be exhilarating for them, but also disorienting, disconcerting, and even frightening. In this chapter, I discuss how you can help your clients adjust to the process of therapy and what to do when they seem reluctant to proceed—reluctant to become of one mind with you and reluctant to experiment with new ways of relating to their problem.

The Latin root of *reluctance* is *luctari,* to struggle. I think of clients' reluctance as their struggle to accept one or more aspects of the therapeutic process, as their way of saying *no* to what doesn't fit for them. Many therapists interpret clients' reluctance as *resistance,* as their neurotic inability to trust the therapeutic relationship, as their stubborn unwillingness to change. They believe that for therapy to be successful, the resistance needs to be broken through or broken down. I take a different tack.[1]

Tanya, twelve, had been living with Tom and Margaret and their daughter Brenda, also twelve, for six months, though she had known them for a few years. Tom and Margaret had become foster parents for the sole purpose of getting custody and adopting Tanya, but now, on the verge of taking the final legal steps, they were beset with second thoughts. Everyone had expected Tanya to take some time to adapt to her new environment, but no one had anticipated her icy refusal to join in family activities and responsibilities. The parents worried about the effect of Tanya's attitude on Brenda, they hated the ever-present tension in the air, and they wondered why they had bothered making such an extraordinary effort to bring her into their family.

The judge overseeing the foster placement and possible adoption was also concerned; he had recommended that the family take Tanya to a family-based inpatient facility, a place where the staff used holding therapy to break through the barriers of emotionally distant children. Tanya's individual therapist supported the judge's position. Having spent two years unsuccessfully trying to "break down her walls," he believed a more intensive approach was necessary to overcome her resistance. Unsure of what to do, the family came to our clinic for advice, and the intake person assigned them to my practicum team.

Partway through the first session, I joined the primary therapist, Alex,[2] in the therapy room for a few minutes so I could tell the family about some villages I had once visited in Greece and Turkey. Built among crumbling structures of earlier civilizations, each village accommodated ancient brick walls in its layout of roads, buildings, and pathways. Rather than tearing such walls down, I told the family, the villagers had protected them for their historic and aesthetic value.

I then expressed my appreciation for the historic and protective importance of Tanya's walls. Given the life she had led and the uncertain future she faced, she would be crazy, I suggested, to let anyone try to dismantle the very things that had been keeping her safe. How frightening to consider taking even one brick off the top of her walls when her hope for a safe and loving family could still be snatched away from her. Of course, Tom and Margaret and Brenda were also scared. They kept looking for the girl they wanted to become one of them, but whenever they sought her out, she was nowhere to be found. Naturally, they wanted Tanya to let them through to her. But what if they looked at her walls differently—say, with the eyes of Greek or Turkish villagers? What if they decided to decorate, rather than destroy, the walls? The idea intrigued them all.

"What color," I asked Tanya, "do you think you should paint your walls?"

"Red."

"Why red?"

"Because it's the color of love."

Alex and I, and I think the family, were surprised and delighted by her answer. Over the next few sessions, we continued to talk about protecting and beautifying these testaments to Tanya's strength and resilience. The parents, the judge, and Tanya's individual therapist had been trying to get her to stop pushing the family (and the therapist) away—trying to separate her from her separating, to negate her efforts to negate them. In contrast, we invited the family to approach Tanya's walls as an integral part of their landscape. Once they did, the walls transformed. The last Alex and I heard, the family had decided not to bother with the inpatient program, and the adoption process was back on track.

From the time we are toddlers, saying *no* is an essential component of our defining our identity: We discover and shape who we are, in part, by defining who we *aren't* and what we *won't* do. So why should your clients abandon this skill the moment they walk into your office? Before they know you, before they trust you, before they know what they're getting themselves in for, they are wise to say *no* to you, keeping themselves separate. Of course, you can't be helpful unless they choose to say *yes* to being in relationship with you and with what you have to offer. Your job is to ensure that they can do so without compromising their integrity, without their needing to say *no*.

When Eric was two, Shelley and I took him to a playground that featured a big wooden contraption, complete with ladders and bridges, slides and stairs. A little girl about Eric's age was prancing on a swinging bridge, and her mother was trying, unsuccessfully, to entice her to get off and accompany her to a shaded picnic area a short distance away, where the father was visiting with friends. As we approached, we heard the mother plead, "Are you ready to get down?"

"No."

"Do you need a drink?"

"No."

"Aren't you hot? You look very hot."

"No."

"Would you like to go see your daddy?"

"No."

"Don't you want to see your daddy?"

"No."

The mother's patience was wearing thin. She wiped the perspiration off her face, made a half-hearted attempt to pluck the little girl off the bridge, and then slumped a little, looking exasperated and defeated. I took a turn.

"Wow, look at you walk across that bridge! And you can climb up those stairs all by yourself!" The little girl marched around, happily. "I can see your mommy. Is that her right there?"

"Yeah!"

"Do you have a daddy, too?"

"Yeah!"

"No, really? You have a daddy?"

"Yeah!"

"*Wow!* You have a *daddy?!*"

"Yeah!"

"Where is your daddy?"

"Right there!" she said, proudly pointing over to the shade.

"*No!* Really? That's your daddy right over there?!"

"Yeah!"

"Are you going to go see your daddy?"

"Yeah!" she said, running over to her mother's arms.

If you are familiar with Milton Erickson's work, you might say that I created a "yes set," asking the little girl questions to which she could happily say *yeah,* and that I saved her the trouble of saying *no* by saying it myself several times. I would describe the interaction somewhat differently. Entering the little girl's world of proud assertion, I phrased my comments and posed my questions so that she could define herself in relation, rather than opposition, to her mother and father, and also, for the duration of our brief conversation, in relation to me. When saying *no* wasn't necessary for her to maintain her integrity, she could say *yeah.* The same is true of clients.

Agreeing to therapy, trusting you, trying hypnosis, venturing change—the people who come to see you can experience these as incredible risks. Once you recognize the potentially high intra- and interpersonal stakes involved for clients committing to a therapeutic relationship, you can explore ways of helping them to relax their struggle, to feel safe and respected enough to let go of their reluctance, to say *yes* (or at least *maybe*) to you, to therapy, to change.

## *When Clients Question Therapy*

Karin and I, both seventeen, had been friends for a couple of years when I realized I had become smitten with her. Boldly (for me), I asked her out on a date, and although she was somewhat taken aback, she agreed. We both had (what I thought to be) a great time, but when I called her the next day with possible plans for the following weekend, she turned me down with a lame excuse. Crushed, I didn't phone her again, and because she lived across town and I had quit the youth orchestra where we'd met, we fell out of touch.

One evening, several years later, when I was back home for Christmas vacation, we got together for dinner. After catching up with each other's news, I asked her how I had, back then, managed to blow it with her. She told me she had found the specificity of my plans unnerving. Here she was still trying to get her head around the idea of our being on a date, and I was busy concretizing our future, explaining that although I could probably only borrow my dad's car one evening a week, I'd be able to ride my bicycle over to her place on Sundays, that I had friends who drove whom we could accompany on weekend hiking trips, that the phone would come in handy for helping each other with homework, that maybe next summer. . . .

You get the idea. Full of plans and full of myself, I was eight steps ahead of her. And this, I think, is the same mistake many of us make with our clients. We leave them in the dust. While they are still questioning whether they are in the right place with the right therapist, we are off, rubbing our hands together, concocting all the ways we'll be able to be helpful. When we get ahead of our clients, we get ahead of ourselves, and we're left wondering why we've got a stuck case. Allow me to offer some ideas for how to back up.

## Think in Terms of Relationship, Rather than Motivation

How motivated are your clients? How much motivation do they have to change? I suppose such questions make a certain amount of sense, given that the Latin root of the word *motivation* is *movere*, to move. Your clients' motivation puts them "into motion," right? But wait. Such a conception implies that your clients actually have a quantity of something inside them—some amount of *motivation*, separate from and prior to their *movement*, that fuels their choices and actions. I'm wary of using such inner abstract entities as explanatory devices because you can so easily start treating them as if they were real, and if you do that, you quickly slide into muddled thinking.[3] If you operate as if your clients have (or are lacking) some level of motivation, you'll then be tempted to use your estimation of this level as the basis for making clinical decisions. Ever asked yourself whether your clients have sufficient motivation to start therapy? Whether they first need to increase it? But how would they go about doing that? How can they increase the amount of an abstraction?

An alternative approach is to think in terms of relationship. Rather than worrying about you clients' inner motivation, attend to how they are *relating or orienting to therapy*. You can do this by listening for the question they are explicitly or implicitly asking you. If they are coming to see you, for example, at the behest of one or more others (family members, the court system, the state, a doctor, a teacher, friends), then the only question they may be asking is, "How do I/we convince you that I/we don't need to be here?" If you're like me, you'll never need convincing. I'm not interested in foisting my services on people who aren't asking for my help.

Some clients *are* asking for help, but they aren't sure about you or about the kind of therapy you are offering. They may be held back by the risks or inconvenience involved in changing, or they may be holding inaccurate assumptions about what you'll be wanting them or not needing them to do—assumptions that may be shutting them down or that will overly restrict your freedom. Whatever the case, you'll want to look for ways of inviting a relationship between them and therapy that opens possibilities for change.

## Invite Involuntary Clients to See You for Reasons of Their Own

When someone other than your clients is responsible for their attending their first session, you will want to figure out to what degree they feel they are there under duress, asking, for example, "If X hadn't told you to come to see me, would you be here today?" If they say *no*, you might follow up with something like this: "If, instead of X *requiring* you to attend the session here, a close friend had *suggested* it, would you have come?" Such questions can help you tease out whether they have any personal stake in sitting in front of you. If they don't, but they're obeying a court order or following a directive from the state's social service agency, you can ask whether they think it would be worth their trouble to explore ways of getting out from under the thumb of whoever is urging or requiring them to see you. In this way, you're inviting them to see therapy as an opportunity rather than as a sentence. If they accept your invitation, you can proceed to help them deal differently with the person or people calling the shots. If they don't, you will do better, following the lead of the MRI folks (e.g., Fisch, Weakland, & Segal, 1982), to work directly (if that's possible) with the person or people who are most concerned about the problem—whoever wants it to change.[4] No use kicking into gear until the person with whom you're talking wants something from you.

## Invite Voluntary Clients with Voluntary Complaints to Commit to Taking Action

A seventy-year-old man, Ed, came to see me, requesting hypnosis to help him quit his fifty-year pack-a-day smoking habit. Unhappily retired for seven years, he talked proudly of his former career and of the office he had had on the sixty-first floor of the Empire State Building. When I discovered that the office had always been maintained as a smoke-free environment, I wondered whether Ed's difficult adjustment to retirement could prove helpful in his becoming a former smoker. If he was still identifying himself in terms of his preretirement life, then perhaps the not-smoking-in-the-office portion of that identity could be vivified and expanded in some way.

I linked the sensation of standing in the elevator of the Empire State Building, moving upward from floor to floor, closer and closer to the office, to the experience of sitting in the comfortable chair in my office, moving down, further and further down, into hypnosis. Later in the session, I told Ed a story of a short young man who went to see Milton Erickson, requesting hypnosis to rectify his arrested physical development. Erickson helped the man develop a new perspective—an ability to see the world as if he were standing one step up on a staircase—and the man subsequently grew six inches.[5] Reasoning that Ed and his lungs might as well benefit from his continuing pride over his former career and the prestigious location of his former office, I said, "If a six-inch change in perspective can release a man's ability to grow, then the enduring memory of a sixty-floor change in perspective can release a man's ability to crave clean air."

Before our second meeting, I got out my calculator and worked out that at a pack a day, Ed had, to date, smoked somewhere in the neighborhood of 365,000 cigarettes. During hypnosis, I described his standing in his Empire State Building office, looking down from his window at dusk, looking down, way down to the ground, where three or four hundred thousand people had gathered, each of them simultaneously lighting up their last cigarette. From that height, I said, he couldn't of course make out individuals, but he *could* see, through the cloud of smoke rising toward him, the glow of the cigarettes.

> And isn't it odd that the way the people are standing, the glow from one-third of a million last cigarettes seems to form individual letters? There's a K . . . there's an N, . . . and an O . . . and another N, . . . and an S, . . . a G, . . . an I, . . . another O, and an M: K . . . N . . . O . . . N . . . S . . . G . . . I . . . O . . . M. And as the cigarettes go up in a last puff of smoke, the letters begin winking out, with just the afterglow left. Now just the memory of the letters, glowing through the smoke, first the N, then the O, then the S, the M, the O, the K, the I, the N, the G, etched there out the window, sixty-one floors down.[6]

Wanting to sprinkle some possibilities for how to say good-bye to a habit that had provided such comfort, I told a variety of stories, one of which was about my son giving up his pacifier habit.

> A few months before he turned three, my son, Eric, agreed with his mother and me that he no longer needed to be bothered sucking on his pacifiers—or, as we called them, his "soothers." Since birth these soothers had been an important part of his life, but they had for some time been more trouble than they were worth. Anytime Eric got upset, he'd say, "I need a soother," but he'd also think he needed one when he felt happy or relaxed. Clearly, *the time had come to let go of the habit*. Together, Eric, his mother, and I came up with a plan for how to say good-bye to something so important. We bought him a new pair of shoes and decided that his stash of remaining soothers would fit comfortably inside the empty box. . . .
>
> My son loved our garbage man. Twice a week before breakfast, hearing the big truck coming down the street, he'd come and grab me, and we'd

dash out the door, waving to the driver and watching the mechanical arm on the side of the truck *effortlessly lift up* the garbage can, turn it upside down, and shake its contents into the center of the truck.

Eric decided that if anyone was going to help him say good-bye to his soothers, it should be his truck-driving friend. The night before our next scheduled pick-up, we lined his shoe box with some paper towels, and we set it carefully on his chest of drawers. Eric's mother wisely decided that *the best time for a ceremonial good-bye is the morning—a time of new beginnings.*

The next day, as we fixed breakfast, Eric walked around with a pacifier so firmly and comfortably planted in his mouth that we wondered whether he had forgotten the plan or had changed his mind. We said nothing, and neither did he. But a little while later, when he heard the distant whine of the approaching garbage truck, Eric reminded us it was *time to take action.* Nestling his three remaining soothers under the paper towel inside the shoe box, he put on the lid, and out we went to the street.

Standing together in front of the garbage can, I asked Eric if he wanted to say good-bye to the soothers before depositing the box inside. *"One last suck,"* he said, taking out each pacifier in turn and placing it in his mouth. After gently, and a little reluctantly, placing them all back in the box, he touched each one in turn, saying, "Bye soother, thanks for the help!" By himself, he put the box in the garbage can, and then ran around the driveway and yard in his new shoes, taking his *first habit-free steps.* His friend the garbage man came and took his pacifiers away. Eric waved and waved good-bye.

I invited Ed to reorient to the therapy room, and we talked about when and how he would smoke his last cigarette. He didn't sound convinced. As he wrote out his check, he said dismissively, "There *is* no thirteenth floor in the Empire State Building, so when you're going up in the elevator, no *thirteen* lights up, and when you're looking out the window on the sixty-first floor, you're only sixty, not sixty-one, floors above the ground."

"Oh, right, of course."

"You see? And anyway, I was only on the sixty-first floor for the last ten or so years of my career. Prior to that, as I told you, I had been on three other floors."

"Uhhuh, yes, I remember."

He then commented on my story of Eric. "Your son wasn't even three when he gave up his pacifiers. He wasn't, see, I'm an old man, and he hadn't been an addict for fifty years. It isn't the same."

A few weeks later, I made a follow-up call, and, as you might guess, I was told the hypnosis had been "a total waste of time and money."

Where did I go wrong? Obviously, I blew it with my description of the Empire State Building, and I miscalculated in telling the story of Eric. But the problem went further. Rushing forward to try to help Ed let go of his cigarettes, I remained so focused on cooking up creative, "individually designed" images and suggestions that I didn't adequately attend to his expectations and concerns. Had I done that, I may have refused or delayed our working together, at least until I got a better sense of his relationship to his habit. It had a grip on him, certainly, but how tightly was he holding onto *it*? If he'd been able to convince me that he was ready to let go, I perhaps could have folded his skepticism and worries into what I said and how I said it, thereby keeping my slips and his dissatisfaction from coming between us.

My failure with this case makes clear that you can invent what you hope to be relevant images and stories of change, but these, in isolation, will never be enough. Clients come to see you, wanting you to do something with their problem, but your job is to help *them* do something with it. Bill O'Hanlon (O'Hanlon & Martin, 1992, pp. 111–119) distinguishes—usefully, I think—between involuntary and voluntary complaints, making the point that hypnosis tends to work great with the involuntary variety (pain, rashes, flashbacks, anxiety, obsessive thinking), but not so great with complaints that involve some degree of deliberate choice (actions that could be demonstrated on request—smoking, yelling, school avoidance, eating too much, bulimia, and so on).

I've had a few people like Ed come to see me—clients who presumed that I would and could "reprogram" them to alter some bothersome or dangerous habit while they reclined, passively accepting a "mind massage." If, as I did with Ed, you fail to adequately challenge this presumption, you're headed for failure. You have to invite your clients to buy into the process of changing, of actively and deliberately making different choices. Hypnosis can be helpful in altering how people orient to the act of choosing, how they experience themselves as they choose, or how they feel once they've made a particular choice, but it can't induce a conscious commitment to change. Ed helped me learn this, helped me alter how I work with clients struggling with a "voluntary complaint."

Bev, a tough, bright divorce lawyer with a gritty sense of humor, called to ask whether hypnosis could help her stop the pack-a-day smoking habit she had acquired ten years earlier while studying for her bar exam. Having just discovered she was pregnant, she felt a sense of urgency about quitting, but she was afraid that if she tried it on her own, she would fail, just like in the past. I told her that despite her desire to quit as soon as possible, our first appointment would have to be for me, not her. Before beginning hypnosis, I said, I would need to ask her a bunch of questions. She agreed, so when we met, I, as promised, asked her about her work and her smoking routines—where, when, and with whom she typically lit up, and which fingers on which hand had become accustomed to holding her cigarettes. Later, we talked about how the ritualized proceedings of a divorce formalize and facilitate the process of ending a relationship. I wondered aloud how she would say good-bye to cigarettes for good. "Will you know as you're smoking it that the cigarette you're holding is your last? Will you have prepared for the ending, or will you only realize after the fact that you won't be lighting up again? Will you keep burning the cigarette all the way to the filter, making sure you suck the last bit of smoke out of it, or will you impatiently stub it out when it's only halfway burned? Or," I said, adopting her descriptive language, "will you take the little fucker and set fire to it, letting it smolder alone for how it has fucked up your lungs and put your baby at risk?"

Just before the end of the session, I suggested that her legal expertise could prove useful for the step she was about to take. She thought for a while and said, "I guess I could create a divorce decree, listing all the grounds for the petition. It seems kind of silly, though." I agreed that from a logical perspective it was pretty ridiculous, but added that her body no doubt would have a different take, given how differently *it* thinks: "You, better than anyone, understand the importance of divorce rituals for marking the end of a relationship and the beginning of a new life. Your body will know how to take such a ritual seriously." As we scheduled her next appointment, we joked about whether and how she could charge for filing the petition.

The following week, Bev presented me with a marvelous official-looking document, a Petition for Dissolution of Marriage, elaborating why the Petitioner (she) was filing for divorce from the Respondent (Camel)—"the Respondent," it said, "has been abusive, . . . has stalked the Petitioner, . . . has caused incessant coughing," and so on. The Petitioner sought "an injunction for protection from the Respondent permanently, . . . allowing the Petitioner a smoke free existence for the remainder of her life." Prior to our beginning hypnosis, Bev signed and dated the petition for both her and her unborn child; I signed as the witness. (And at the end of the session, she wrote on the "memo" line of the check that the amount was to cover the petition filing fee.)

Bev's petition served as the foundation for our hypnotic work. She had spoken earlier of her concern about the physical sensations of nicotine withdrawal, so I addressed this in what I suggested:

> Those fingers on your right hand can remember as I'm speaking what it felt like to hold and light a cigarette, . . . but they can also remember typing and signing your decree. And as your body begins to notice the absence of nicotine, you will begin to feel the vibrations of freedom, freedom from the Respondent, and those penholding fingers can send those vibrations all the way through your body, can send the memory of signing the petition all the way through your body, giving you the distinct taste of freedom, giving you a vibrating massage of freedom. And won't it be so interesting in twenty years for you to have a conversation with your child? A conversation where you express your gratitude for the inspiration to sign your way to freedom.
>
> Those fingers that hold your pen, those fingers can provide you with a signature way of freeing you from that last cigarette, allowing you some perspective, allowing you to reconnect with your self, your surroundings, your baby. Your fingers can give you a signature experience of freedom, that automatic signing-your-name freedom, sending an automatic feeling through your whole body.

I took Bev forward in time to a stressful event and offered her the opportunity to feel how her fingers could "send a jolt of pride, accomplishment, and astonishment, a signature burst of freedom, the signature experience of defining a new beginning, vibrating through your body, creating a ripple effect through your days and evenings and nights and mornings and weeks and hours and months and years to come." I described someone offering her a cigarette to help her deal with her child having a high fever or to cope with someone important dying (she had recently dealt with the deaths of close friends and family members), and I suggested that when that happened, she allow her body to feel disoriented, confused as to why a cigarette would even presume to think she'd be remotely interested in its fake comfort.

During a follow-up conversation six months later, Bev told me she had left my office feeling happily elated and hadn't "given cigarettes another thought."

### Provide Fence-sitting Clients with an Opportunity, but not a Push, to Get Down

Sometimes, clients aren't so much saying *no* to therapy as they are saying *I don't know.* A fence-sitting orientation holds more promise for your being able to do something useful—your clients might, after all, warm up to the idea of therapy. But if you try to nudge them to get off the fence, and particularly if you encourage them to jump down on your side of it, then the only way they can assert their independence is to say *no* to you. If, instead, you support their making their decision in their own time and in their own way, you make it possible for them to maintain their sense of identity *and* to choose to work with you.

A seventy-five-year-old woman from Boston, visiting her daughter in Florida, came to see me a few weeks before she was scheduled to fly home. The daughter, worried about her mother's arthritis and diabetes and high cholesterol, had urged her to try hypnosis as a way of controlling her pain and her diet. But the mother, Amy, had her doubts about all doctors and all treatments. She told me that for most of her life she had "gone along with the crowd," but for the last ten years, since becoming diabetic and since her arthritis had worsened, she no longer cared "about fitting in." Before, she always "looked after everyone else first," but now she prioritized her own needs, and that meant "being her own person" and doing what she wanted, despite what her doctors, husband, and daughter advised: "I defy my doctors, and if my husband tries to tell me what to eat, I defy him, too. I cheat like hell on my diet. If I want candy, I'm going to have it."

I told her I respected her doubts about coming to see me, and I warned her, "Hypnosis may not be helpful. Your coming here could turn out to be a complete waste of your time and money." By my saying it, she didn't have to. I then went on to elaborate the various ways she might be disappointed:

Even if the hypnosis *is* helpful, you may notice only minor relief. You might notice a change in your experience of your arthritis but no change in how you go about choosing what to eat. Or you might find yourself eating differently while your arthritis continues pretty much the same. Of course, it is possible you will experience moderate or even significant benefits, but you might not notice them right away. You may recognize the difference only gradually, not until after you return to Boston. But you know how difficult it is to notice something that isn't there. I remember getting a bunch of stuff stolen out of my apartment when I was in graduate school, and it took me weeks and weeks to realize the extent of what was gone. How are you supposed to notice things that are no longer there? How do you notice the *absence* of pain or the *not eating* of certain foods? Unless you're like my wife, who remembers the way renovated houses in our neighborhood looked prior to their changes, you might just get used to things being different without being able to put your finger on what's changed. Things might improve for you, but you'll think back to coming here and chalk it up as a waste.

By highlighting the possibility of Amy's ignoring or discounting any possible benefits of our working together, I was able to simultaneously protect her ability to be her own person *and* elaborate several ways change might occur: The change might be only minor; it might occur in one area of concern but not the other; it might be more significant, but then only be noticed gradually or not at all.

Amy agreed that seeing me might be a waste, or that even if it weren't, she might never recognize the benefits. We went on to talk about the importance of defiance. Her father had died, she told me, when she was nine, and her mother "was a saint," so she hadn't, until the last ten years or so, had that wonderful teenager pleasure of defying authority. She now knew that given the choice of "being good" (i.e., following her diet, following her doctor's advice, doing what she was told) and "being bad" (not letting others tell her what to do), she would always choose the "bad" option. A "good Catholic," she believed that if God were to frown on sweets, then she would try harder, but she thought he probably wasn't too concerned, and she knew he appreciated her lack of vanity. I suggested that her defiance must surely be a way of showing respect for God, given that God must look kindly on anyone fighting for integrity. I then told her about how caffeine dependent I had felt back in my early twenties, about how I got so I needed to keep refueling myself with coffee every few hours. Finally I decided I wasn't going to let caffeine limit what I could and couldn't do—I didn't want a mere substance calling the shots. How liberating it was to refuse to be ordered around.

At the end of the appointment, Amy decided, on her own, to return the following week for a two-hour hypnosis session. It went well, and four months later, her daughter called to say that her mother was "doing great—much better than before." I helped create a relationship with Amy that allowed her to retain—to celebrate— her defiant spirit, but because I didn't dole out any advice, she didn't find it necessary to turn that spirit against me. She was able, instead, to use it to defy the people and substances in her life that needed to be put in their place.

## When Clients Question You

I've supervised many new therapists over the years, and most have worried about what to do if and when their clients start questioning their competence and credentials. "What should I do," they ask me, "if a couple wants to know how old I am, whether I'm married, and if I have children? Or what my degree is and how many cases I've seen? Do I tell them that I'm only twenty-three, have never dated anyone longer than a year, and have no desire to have children? Do I reveal that, God help them, they are my first guinea pigs? Should I warn them that I've only got a lousy bachelor's degree and haven't a clue what I'm doing?"

If you get it in your head that you can't be helpful as a therapist until you're a middle-aged, happily married parent with thousands of client-contact hours under your belt, you're sunk. With such a belief, what are your options? Misrepresent who you are? Introduce yourself to all new clients with an apology for your age and inexperience? Thank them for putting up with your incompetence? I still, at forty-five (and happily married with kids and all those client-contact hours under my belt), sometimes get grilled, and my answers don't always satisfy.

Some clients *will* question you. Expect it. Get over it. Relish it. Here are some ideas for how to respond when your clients turn up the heat.

### Avoid Personas

Lori, a twenty-four-year-old woman with the fresh-faced appearance of a mature teenager, was talking with a middle-aged couple about their fourteen-year-old daughter. Considering that this was the first session of her first case, Lori was doing remarkably well, asking great questions and listening attentively. But every so often she would sit up straight in her chair and make an official-sounding pronouncement about the business of parenting or the social lives of teenagers. The couple seemed to be taking her mini-lectures in stride, but I, watching from behind the one-way mirror, was concerned that the husband was tuning her out and questioning her credibility. During our post-session discussion, I joked with Lori about the times she seemed to be talking with an upper-class English accent, and I asked her what was going on.

Lori was concerned about her youthful appearance, and she wanted to be taken seriously. Not yet sure how to present herself as a therapist, she was offering the couple her best impersonation of a seasoned professional. I told her that the self-conscious attempt to adopt a "therapist persona" is probably the fastest way to convince clients not to trust you. If you don't trust yourself, why should they? When she stopped trying to be someone other than who she was, Lori was able to get down to the business of actually being a therapist, and the husband ended up accepting her and her suggestions.

### Take an "I'm-not-Invested-in-Your-Sticking-with-Me" Position

In her first session with a loud, angry couple, a therapist in my practicum, Kristy, offered an empathic paraphrase of what her clients had been telling her. A soft-spoken woman, Kristy probably sounded more tentative in her statement than she actually was, but the clients responded negatively. They dismissed her efforts as incompetent, derisively questioning her credentials and speaking to her like she was an idiot. Holding her composure, and knowing she couldn't proceed with therapy as long as her clients were concerned about her ability to help, Kristy explained that she wanted to take a short break to consult with her colleagues. When she came behind the mirror, one of the team members suggested that when she returned to the therapy room, she adopt what the MRI folks call a "one-down position" (Fisch, Weakland, & Segal, 1982), apologizing for her poor performance and explaining that she gets rattled when people are screaming. Kristy said she wouldn't feel comfortable doing this, so we decided, instead, that she would thank the clients for helping to keep her on track and would offer to refer them to another therapist if they were concerned she wouldn't be able to help them. This fit for her, and when she returned to the therapy room, she talked to the clients with considerable poise and sincerity. No doubt recognizing her confident and nondefensive tone, they declined her offer to refer them to someone else. Instead of taking a one-down position, Kristy took an "I'm-not-invested-in-your-sticking-with-me" position.

You may not meet your clients' specifications of an ideal (or even an adequate) therapist, but as long as you're comfortable with your (perceived) limitations and you don't get caught up trying to convince your clients to trust or respect you, you can figure out together whether they would do best finding another therapist. If they decide to stay, you can treat their decision as a vote of confidence and move on to addressing the problem that prompted them to contact you in the first place.

## Match Your Clients' Level of Intensity and Formality

It's not that I think the ability to say *fuck* is an essential therapeutic skill. Indeed, I know excellent therapists who never utter the word in professional conversations, and perhaps not even in private ones. But if your clients live and think inside an earthy vocabulary, if they talk about "getting a hard-on," "getting wet," "getting pissed off," or "scoring good shit," then you risk being written off if, in your follow-up questions and comments, you use phrases such as "developing an erection," "achieving lubrication," "becoming irritated," or "procuring good-quality illegal substances." Euphemisms and other niceties can convince your clients that you're too proper to trust—or, more to the point, that you don't know shit. One of my supervisees once worked with a woman who, as she herself put it, "slept around" more than she thought wise. The therapist asked her to describe to him how she felt after making love. The woman looked at him long and hard before replying, icily, "I don't 'make love' with guys. I *fuck* them."

Another supervisee, Tommie, an experienced clinician from South Carolina, liked my suggestion to loosen up her word choices (or, as I put it, to practice "fuck" therapy), but she had a hard time getting her tongue to shake off its genteel Southern upbringing. Several months after completing my practicum, though, she came up to me in our training clinic, handed me a tape of a session she had conducted the night before with a couple, and encouraged me to watch the portion she had cued up. Here's what I heard:

WIFE: I used to be affectionate with him, but it's a big hassle, it's a pain in the ass. I don't want to put the effort into it.

TOMMIE: So when Jeff is being a pain in the ass, what can you do to cause him not to be a pain in the ass?

HUSBAND: Leave me alone.

W: Is that what I do?

T: Does it work?

H: Leave me alone. Yeah.

W: Sort of. But let me tell you something. Do you know what happened? Friday, I lost it. He said something to me like only he can, and I told him to fuck himself. And I *screamed* at him. . . .

T: So Jeff, what did you do when she said, "Fuck you!"?

W: He told me to go fuck myself, too. But then do you know what he did? He went into the room, I came out, and he acted like a different person. He likes when I actually act like this. . . . He respects it. . . . Now I was pissed.

Tommie's word choices flowed like honey from her tongue, helping to reassure the couple that they didn't need to shield her from the blood and guts of their relationship.

The complementary side of this suggestion is also important. You and your sexual partner may, in the privacy of your own vocabulary, "fuck your brains out," but if your clients "make love" or "engage in sexual intercourse," then while you're talking with them about their understanding of their sexual relationship, you'll want to adopt *their* descriptions, not impose yours.[7]

## When Clients Question Hypnosis

When I was in my early twenties, near the beginning of my study of tai chi chuan, one of the more senior students in my club asked me if I would like him to use hypnosis to help me advance my skills more quickly. I declined his offer, whereupon he congratulated me for having the wisdom and determination to learn the "right" (read, "slow") way. He explained that had I chosen to "submit" to his "hypnotic will," I would have weakened my own "willpower" to withstand other, possibly negative, influences in the future. A few years later, after I had done some reading and taken a hypnosis workshop or two, I was able to articulate clearly the student's mistaken assumptions, but at the time, I was a bit spooked by what he said.

With such misinformed people spouting off; with all the hypno-entertainers on television and stage demonstrating how they can compel people to make fools of themselves; with all the B-grade suspense movies portraying hypnotists as all-powerful, and often evil, mind-controllers; and with all the cheesy newspaper and yellow-pages ads for miraculous hypnosis cures, I'm amazed that *anyone* makes it into my office with a positive, reasonable view of hypnotherapy. You can thus expect most of your clients to come in with at least some inaccurate assumptions about the work you do. Clearing these up will help allay many concerns,[8] but you never want to be in the position of trying to *convince* clients to become of one mind with you.

### Encourage Clients to Make a
### Personal, Informed Choice

Some years ago, a psychiatrist referred a woman to me who was suffering from panic attacks. The client, Susan, hadn't driven for some months and had been avoiding malls, restaurants, and grocery stores, as well as escalators and elevators. During the first session I asked her what the psychiatrist had told her about me—had she mentioned that I practiced hypnosis? She had indeed, but Susan wasn't sure she wanted to try it. A couple of close friends, influenced by the teachings of their conservative religion, had warned her of its dangers. They had told Susan a story of a woman who had gone to a hypnotist with a fear of heights; at the end of treatment, the woman was not only still afraid of high places, but this fear had also extended to many other places and activities. Although Susan did not embrace all of her friends' religious convictions, she *had* been swayed by their horror story and was, as a result, nervous about the possibility of trying hypnosis. In addition, her recent divorce—her husband had left her for another woman—and some negative experiences with previous male therapists had soured her on the prospect of being helped by a man. Susan's most recent therapist had attempted hypnosis a few times, but she hadn't trusted him and nothing of consequence had come of it. Sizing him up as "a flake," she had gone back to her psychiatrist for a referral to a different therapist. By the time she arrived at my office, she was understandably edgy.

I answered all of Susan's preliminary questions, some probing, some less so—yes, I'm happily married; no, I've never been divorced; yes, I think hypnosis could be helpful—and after hearing of her experiences, I agreed she had some excellent reasons for not trusting me and for avoiding hypnotherapy. "Given the beliefs and practices of some of the people claiming to offer hypnotherapy," I said, "I don't blame pastors for urging their congregations to stay away from hypnotists altogether. And given your personal experience with the flake you just saw, you obviously have some excellent reasons for listening to your friends."

"But," she countered, "Lindsay [her eighteen-year-old daughter] told me to ignore them. She read about hypnosis in her freshman psychology class, and she says I need to give it a chance. So now I don't know what to do." I told her a story about one of my students, a Christian minister, who, despite his apprehension, had volunteered for a demonstration in my hypnosis class at the university and had been rewarded with a pleasant and deeply relaxing experience. "But then," I cautioned, "this may not be relevant to you, given that he is a man and had known me for a long time, first."

Recognizing that Susan felt pulled in opposite directions by her daughter and her friends, I proposed she bring them all to her next appointment. This would allow them to speak their minds, allow me to clear up any mistaken understandings, and allow Susan to figure out where she stood. She refused my proposal, but she did agree that, since she would be the one choosing to try or not try hypnosis, it made sense for her to listen not only to others' views, but also to her own. Providing her with some straightforward information about what hypnosis is and how it works, I suggested she take a week to tease out *her* concerns and *her* hopes and to come back with further questions. When she returned for her next appointment, she told me she had decided to give hypnosis a try. A month or two later, following some successful work together, she had the serendipitous pleasure of meeting one of her hypnosis-fearing friends on the escalator at a local mall. When the woman expressed surprise at seeing her in such a seemingly panic-inducing place, Susan mentioned in an offhand manner that she had just come from her hypnotherapist's office and was on her way to a restaurant to have lunch with her daughter.

If you've read and thought enough about hypnosis to be able to give an extemporaneous layperson's explanation of what it is and how it works, then you will be able to help most clients form reasonable expectations about what's possible. But if your ability to describe hypnosis goes out the window when you're put on the spot, you would do well to prepare some written descriptions your clients can read.[9]

## Take an "I'm-not-Invested-in-Your-Trying-Hypnosis" Position

Some clients come to their first appointment confident you will work miracles, unconcerned about who you are, what you don't know, or how you work; others, arriving with the certainty (or at least the strong suspicion) that you can do nothing to help them, will be ready to find some reason to doubt your therapeutic capacity. Either expectation can pull you into responding with excessive encouragement: "Oh sure, of course I can relieve you of your problem!" or "Don't write me off yet! I know, if you'll only give me the chance, that I'll be able to help you!" I neither try to live up to clients' overly optimistic hope nor try to quell their overly pessimistic doubt. Instead, I do my best to fashion some uncertainty about what will or can happen, to create some anticipation for the unanticipated.

A colleague, Arlene, had been seeing Keith and his wife Miki for marital and (with their son) family therapy, and although they were all pleased with several positive changes, Arlene was concerned that Keith's chronic back pain and daily migraines were getting in the way of further progress. Badly hurt in a car accident a year and a half earlier, Keith had undergone surgeries in both his back and neck, but they had only been partially successful. Most days, Keith's headache kept him from being able to think straight, and it and his back kept him from returning to renovating houses. For ten years, he'd had steady and well-paying work refurbishing older homes, but his doctors were advising him not to even consider tackling the physical demands of roofing, drywalling, carpentry, and so on.

When Arlene first recommended that Keith come to see me for hypnosis, he refused to consider the possibility, despite (or, perhaps, in part because of) Miki's enthusiastic encouragement. Hopeless about his future, fatigued by the pain, and fed up with his doctors, he wasn't interested in yet another disappointment. But Arlene patiently continued to talk about hypnosis and me, and Miki continued to plead, and eventually Keith decided to come in for an initial visit—though probably more as a way to appease his wife than to satisfy any curiosity. I invited Miki and Arlene to join Keith in the session, and the four of us talked for an hour and a half about Keith's accident, the way he had been spending his days, what the doctors and Miki had been telling him, what measures he had taken in response to the pain, and what he had noticed as far as variations in the sensations—times when they got worse and times when they weren't as bad. We also talked about his understanding of hypnosis (mostly informed by what he'd seen on television) and my way of using hypnosis for pain. Near the end of our time together, I asked Keith and Miki if either of them had any additional concerns they wanted to bring up.

MIKI: Is there anything he [Keith] can think about, about being
    hypnotized or about, you know, when you started talking about
    roofing and plumbing and the electrical
DOUGLAS: Yeah.
M: work he does, and you saw how he went "ha! hmm hmm!" [makes
    a face] when you talked about that and dealing with the pain and

hypnosis. Is there anything he can *think* about to try to open himself up to hypnosis?

From what I've told you of the couple's interactions, you no doubt can recognize what a mistake it would have been for me to have blithely offered some "helpful hints" for how Keith could counteract his skepticism.

D: I don't think people should *try* to open themselves up to anything.
M: No?

Trying to believe in something is like trying to be happy: The concerted effort undermines the goal. This is because neither belief nor happiness is an object that can be reached for and grasped; both are ways of orienting, and, as such, they can't be directly obtained.

D: It's like, [to Keith] when you'd be asked to solve an electrical or
   plumbing or roof problem, and you'd have to write up an estimate
   of what all needed doing, you were never willing to commit yourself
   to anything until you could see where the problem was and until
   you could get your hands on it. I think it would be a mistake for me
   to try to convince you of anything until you start actually
   recognizing that something has changed. Why the hell should you
   believe anything I say? You've never met me before, and you don't
   know anything about hypnosis except for all the bogus people you
   said you've seen on television, so I *certainly* wouldn't want you to go
   away and try to believe in me or believe in hypnosis.

By acknowledging the legitimacy of Keith's misgivings (connecting to his separation from hypnosis), I freed him up to venture a more positive assessment. I also encouraged his hands-on method of learning—only when he had tried hypnosis and noticed changes should he consider giving it any credibility.

KEITH: I heard some good things. I mean I've heard both sides. Her
   [Miki's] brother-inlaw—
M: Yeah, he quit smoking,
K: For about what? Twenty some years.
M: Yeah, almost twenty years.

I didn't know whether he respected his brother-in-law, and I suspected that quitting smoking might seem trivial to him, relative to his dealing with his pain. I thus continued to encourage his critical intelligence.

D:  Well, what really matters is what happens to *you*. What *I* believe is that when you start noticing something changing, then you'll get on board. And why should you get on board before? So, no [to Miki], I don't think he should go home and squeeze his eyes shut and try. . .

Miki took exception to my comment,

M:  No, I don't mean that, I don't mean that.

But Keith responded to it with the very curiosity she had been hoping for.

K:  Is meditation anything like it?
D:  Well, it's very similar in some important ways.

Keith told me about how he had, at times, "meditated" while sitting in his truck, parked under a tree and staring at a lake. He'd found that this had sometimes helped "clear his head" of the pain. Knowing that he had picked up many of his construction skills on the job, I underscored how he had, all on his own, figured out how to do a form of self-hypnosis, so that all we'd probably be doing is helping him fine-tune and expand on the meditation he already knew how to do. He and Miki returned for a few subsequent appointments, and he experienced significant pain relief from the hypnosis we did and the daily self-hypnosis he implemented.[10] This wouldn't have happened had I joined Miki in trying to *convince* Keith to trust me, to believe in hypnosis, to abandon his skepticism—I'm sure he would never have returned for a second appointment.

## *When Your Clients Ask for Help You Can't or Won't Give Them*

I still recall the astonished pleasure I felt when I first realized I could liberate myself from other people's social expectations. Relational freedom! Long before I became a therapist, I was standing on a street corner in Vancouver, British Columbia, waiting for a light to change, when a young woman stepped in front of me. "Hi there!" she said, "Are you new in town?" I had been daydreaming, so I was a little startled by her forthright question. I looked at her for a moment, silently wondering which cult she was recruiting for. I must have looked blank a little too long. "Do you speak English?" she inquired, brightly.

Again I paused, wondering what had inspired her question. Did I look like a Quebecker? A European? Should I try out my French? My silent musings were interrupted by her next question. "Parlez-vous Français?" she asked, sounding like she'd just arrived from Montreal.

Relieved I hadn't tried faking her out with a mumbled "Je ne parle pas Anglais," I weighed various possible responses in my head, but my thought processes were much slower than her tongue. Exasperated, she demanded, "Well what language *do* you speak, then?"

At this point my self-developed fluency in gobbledygook came to the rescue. "Cos tebiento von chetas. Neekta pan sorruto. Hikeh blotos?"

"So you don't understand what I'm saying? What language is that?"

I smiled. "Corrutona? Hostos munchess?" This was enough for her. The light changed; she stayed put; I walked away, cult-free. I had, quite by accident, discovered how to slip out of the constraints of social politeness, realizing, for instance, that questions don't necessarily need to be answered. This has proved invaluable in the therapy room (and at car dealerships); however, since I am interested in maintaining a *connected* separation with clients, I don't speak gobbledygook or blurt out non sequiturs or act weirdly (okay, not *too* weirdly), and I don't walk away from them. I do attempt to enter their experience *and* remain free to respond creatively to what we talk about and what they ask of me. If my clients and I are going to cook up intraventive solutions together, I need to be at liberty to be of one mind with them *and* keep in touch with my sense of play, humor, and mischief, as well as my understanding of how concordance and therapeutic change happen.[11]

Connecting well with clients is particularly important because you often have to disappoint them. They come to see you, hoping you will help them change what's bugging them, and your job is to respond to their request without being constrained by their expectations. Frequently, the way they are setting out to solve their problem is the very thing that's getting in their way, so if you were to give them exactly what they wanted, you'd only be contributing to their unworkable solution attempts.[12] You thus must walk a line. If you attempt to give them just what they're requesting, you will likely fail to be helpful. But if you don't satisfy their request, you risk irritating, offending, or dissatisfying them. And although you don't want to be constrained by their agenda, neither do you want simply to negate it and impose your own. You have to respect their requests for help *and* respect the necessity of keeping your options open, of feeling free to be intraventively inventive. When you walk this line successfully, when you manage to maintain both a connection to and a connected separation from your clients, you won't be giving them precisely what they expected, but their initial disappointment will fade as their predicament resolves.

## Anticipate Imminent Change

One of my clients wanted the security of a standing appointment. Dissatisfied with my practice of booking the next week's meeting at the end of the current one, he wanted me to schedule him at least a month's worth of appointments in advance. I acknowledged his needing to know that I would be available to see him, but I was concerned, I said, that such an arrangement could create the implicit assumption that significant shifts in his problem were unlikely to be imminent. I'm always anticipating that change, if not already underway, is just around the corner, and I didn't want the scheduling of advance appointments to dull my client's ability to recognize when something new was happening. We agreed to book two or three sessions at a time, with the provision that we would assess and decide each time we met whether the next appointment was necessary. I wanted both of us to have the option, I said, to cancel an already scheduled session if it looked like some nascent change needed time to develop.

## Adopt the Professional Sensibility
## of Mary Poppins

At the funeral for one of his close friends, a psychiatrist went up to the deceased's thirty-year-old daughter and, after offering his condolences, pressed two prescriptions into her palm, one for sleep-

ing pills, the other for an antidepressant. He told her that the
medications would help her through the difficult weeks and months
ahead, and he urged her to find a therapist for her inevitable depression. She didn't immediately fill the prescriptions, but, following the
psychiatrist's advice regarding therapy, she called me for an appointment. At the beginning of the first session, she told me she anticipated needing weekly appointments for six to nine months. Asked
how she had come up with this time frame, she explained that this
was how long she imagined she'd be feeling depressed.

We talked about her grief over her mother's death, but also about
the rest of her life—her career, close friends, activities, and so on. She
seemed to me to be responding amazingly well, given the circumstances, so I asked how she thought I could be helpful. She looked at
me quizzically and said, "You're the professional—don't you know?"
I told her that in contrast to her mother's friend, I differentiate between depression and grief, and I don't assume that deep sadness necessarily requires medication and professional involvement. "My expertise," I said, "doesn't reside in knowing what's best for you, but,
rather, in helping you discover what you already know and are able to
learn. I help people who are stuck, but I don't get the sense you are.
You're grieving, but I don't assume that this means there's something
wrong with you. How could you feel otherwise?"

By the end of the session, the woman decided that perhaps she
didn't need to schedule a series of appointments. I saw her, at her
request, a few weeks later and once again a month or so after that. She
mourned deeply her mother's death, withdrawing for a while from
some aspects of her busy life, but she never found it necessary to rely
on the medication, and she decided that she didn't require a professional to guide her. I didn't give her what she originally requested, but
I did manage to convey my trust in her ability to move through her
experience in a meaningful way. This is such an important gift you can
give your clients—the idea that they have the strength and perspicac-
ity not to need you to accompany them through difficult times.

I'm happy to schedule appointments when my clients and I agree
that doing so might prove helpful, but I tell them in the first session
that I'm in the business of putting myself out of business, that I
prefer to get the hell out of their lives as soon as they're headed in a
direction that works for them. Like Mary Poppins, I only want to
"stay until the wind changes."

## Leave Coaching to Coaches

A woman I once knew, Jennifer, told me about an eventful dinner she had had with a former boyfriend. He had taken her to an upscale restaurant, where they ordered an exquisite bottle of wine, an exotic appetizer, and expensive entrees. He then left the table for fifteen or twenty minutes, reappearing long after the wine had been poured and the appetizer had stopped being appetizing. Jennifer, none too nicely, asked him where he'd been. After a tense silence, he admitted that he had been on the phone to his therapist, getting up-to-the-minute advice and support. Wrong answer. "Advice? Support? For what!?" she demanded. "For how to ask you to marry me. For how to show you this," he said, producing an engagement ring from his pocket. Wrong answer. Predicting that he would probably be needing to dash to the phone booth in the middle of their wedding ceremony (cell phones hadn't yet been invented), Jennifer refused the ring and broke off the relationship.

Unlike Jennifer's boyfriend's therapist, I don't provide an on-call, in-the-moment coaching service for clients in the midst of important life events. I'm happy to help them prepare themselves for anxiety-provoking situations, but I don't want to be an intimate part of their experiences and relationships. They deserve better. They need be able to know, in the moment and upon reflection, that responsibility for their choices and actions belongs to *them*.

## Be Willing to Call it Quits

I love going to great movies, but I enjoy almost as much walking out of lousy ones. I always give the actors and production people the benefit of the doubt for twenty minutes or so, but if the movie doesn't measure up, if it doesn't manage to grab me in some way, I cut my losses and leave. Liberation!

I'm a more patient therapist than movie-goer, but I'm never complacent. If my clients and I don't seem to be getting anywhere, I'm usually the first to broach the possibility of our stopping or at least breaking for a while.[13] I don't want to be taking their money if our work together isn't making a difference.

I'm not suggesting you threaten your clients—"you've got fifteen minutes to come up with a satisfactory goal, or I'll send you home"; "change in the next three sessions or I'll refuse to see you anymore"—and you'll do best if you approach therapeutic process as an opportunity for collaboration. But you also don't want your clients to be thinking that you're scheduling their next appointment for your monetary, rather than their therapeutic, benefit. If, despite your best efforts, you aren't (or are no longer) helping, then stopping is both ethical and responsible. Underscore your clients' strengths and potential, apologize for your limitations, give them the option of coming back in the future, offer to make a referral to someone else, and help them appreciate that saying no to therapy can be a way of saying yes to themselves.

I saw Rachel for many more sessions than is common for me. She liked and respected me, and I was confident she would find a way out of the stagnant place she had found herself. Fed up with her job, living arrangements, and the aesthetic wasteland of her surroundings, she wanted desperately to move, but she didn't have the financial security to make a sudden decision and, besides, she didn't want just to bolt. She struggled to find a sense of meaning and a purpose to keep going, and I did my best to offer a respectful counterpoint to her laments. Over the course of our sessions, she started walking regularly, began actively looking for job transfers, stopped using her bed as a safe haven during the day, and explored possibilities of going back to school. Still, after numerous sessions, her life hadn't taken off in a new direction, and she remained, overall, dissatisfied with therapy.

One day she came in and said she wasn't sure she was getting anything out of seeing me. I congratulated her on what I saw as a life-affirming assessment, underscoring that therapy is often an overrated activity. If I wasn't helping her accomplish her goals, then, I said, she might more wisely invest her time in art classes and her money in a financial planner.

Four months later I called to do a follow-up. In the time since we'd stopped our sessions, she had managed to land two serious job offers in other parts of the country. The first she turned down, despite her interest in the company, because she found the owners too chauvinist. The second looked much better, and she was weighing her options. In addition, she'd met a man online two months earlier and was, for the first time in years, seriously considering the possibility of getting involved. I said, "Just look at what happens when you're smart enough to fire your therapist!"

I always worry when I contact clients for follow-up information that hearing from me will prompt them to once again seek therapy. I was thus concerned when, a few days later, Rachel called, sounding anxious and wanting to talk.[14] I asked her what was going on, and she told me that she'd received a message four hours earlier from an executive in the second company with which she had interviewed. He was offering her the position and wanted her to get back to him immediately. She said she felt frozen; she hadn't returned the call yet, and she didn't know if she should take the job. I asked her what seemed to be holding her back. Although she had several concrete reservations, the primary sticking point was the nausea she was feeling at having to make such a momentous decision.

As I had in some of our sessions, I distinguished between two sorts of fear—the solid kind that you should listen to and the translucent kind that can be walked through. Often, I said, your body can't tell the difference—in both cases you may well feel nauseated, chilled, tight, and short of breath. The solid kind can help you avoid making a serious mistake, such as when your fear of falling keeps you from getting too close to the edge of a cliff. The translucent kind, if you mistake it as solid, can keep you from taking important steps, can send you back under the covers, attempting to find safety. But if you can recognize translucent fear for what it is, you can walk through it, like when you don't let your fear of messing up keep you from rising to a challenge.

A few days later, Rachel came back for a final appointment. She had returned the executive's call and accepted the position, and she was now preparing to move within three weeks. No longer feeling trapped, she didn't find our city and the people in it to be nearly as oppressive as in the past. In fact, she talked with regret about individuals, activities, and places she would miss. I reiterated my admiration for how she had created and prepared for the possibility of such a significant change *after* leaving therapy.

## Think Like a Contrarian, Offering Intraventive Mischief Rather than Interventive Rescuing

I once saw a creative couple who described themselves as "contrarians." Whenever someone they didn't like told them what to do, they did the opposite, and whenever they were confronted with an intractable problem, they would imagine what it would look like if they turned it upside down, backwards, or inside out, or if they reversed it in time. With my longstanding interest in Taoism (inspired, no doubt, by my contrary nature), I was enchanted by their dialectical thought process, as well as the label they put on it: "Contrarian" describes beautifully my inclinations whenever a person anxiously tells me that he or she (or I) *must* do something and *must* do it *immediately*. I'm always visited by the nice, slow contrarian thought, "Hmm. Really? How interesting. I wonder what would and could happen if for some reason you (or I) did something different, maybe even the opposite of what you want?"

Imagine a client coming to you, fearful of her visions. She tells you about evil spirits from another dimension who have been lurking about, spirits who seem to want to enter her body through her mouth. She finds them frightening but also, somehow, alluring. She asks you to use hypnosis to construct a kind of psychic force-field, strong enough to repulse the spirits and send them tumbling back to their own dimension. How would you orient to her request? What suggestions would you develop?

A therapist once approached me regarding his work with such a client. Wary himself of "dark forces in the universe" and thus unnerved by her visions, he had strongly advised the woman, prior to talking with me, to mount a resolute defensive campaign. He was particularly disturbed, he said, by what he considered her "perverse attraction" to the spirits, so he had admonished her not to "let them come anywhere near" her. Frightened at the prospect of his client (or anyone) "messing with the dark side of the spirit world," he was looking for ways to use hypnosis to help her erect a protective barrier.

I wondered aloud about what would happen if the woman were to continue her unrelenting heroic efforts. Since part of her found the spirits alluring, she would need to continue battling not only the spirits themselves, but also her inclination to relax her vigilance. Surely this would prove to be impossibly exhausting. Was there not another, an intraventive, way of achieving safety? What if the therapist, when his client told him she felt pulled to swallow the evil spirits, said "Oh cool!" to himself,[15] instead of "Oh my God, no!"? What if he thought like a contrarian?

I told the therapist that I considered the woman's inclination to swallow the spirits to be anything but perverse; rather, I thought it a brilliant inspiration. Was her digestive system not perfectly designed for protecting her from dark forces? Her stomach and intestines would no doubt know how to transform and use anything from the spirits that proved to be nutritious (i.e., valuable), and they would also know how to treat as fiber anything that couldn't properly be digested. Thus, it seemed to me the woman already knew the best—that is, the safest and most creative—way to deal with the spirits. All she had to do was follow her gut reaction: swallow the spirits, allow her body to digest what it could, and then let it eliminate the roughage.

Talk about swallowing—the therapist had been swallowed up by his client's fears, and his efforts had thus been rescue-oriented: He had been trying to save her from evil and from herself. When your clients are desperate—frightened, exhausted, in pain, fed up—you may find yourself pulled into interventive crisis mode, scrambling for separative solutions. But if you are to become an insider *and* maintain your relational freedom, you will need to respond associationally, not dissociationally, to their dilemmas. That's what they're paying you for.

Bernice, a forty-year old accountant, made ongoing, unsuccessful efforts to keep the world from irritating her. Nothing lined up as neatly as the columns in her databases, and so her vigilant efforts to organize her environment had left her exhausted and miserable. We were a few minutes into our third hypnosis session when she suddenly opened her eyes and told me she needed to adjust the position of her chair. The furniture in the office was arranged in such a way that we weren't quite facing each other, and this "lack of alignment" felt too uncomfortable for her to proceed with trance.

As she stood up to move her chair, I, visited by some contrarian mischief, asked her if she would be willing to try an experiment. She tentatively agreed. I suggested she sit back down in the "out of alignment" position, allow her eyes to close again, and prepare herself to learn something significant. As she slowly lowered herself into her seat, she began to cry.

BERNICE: It feels like a pressure. I'm facing this way, and you're over there, so your voice comes at me obliquely. It needs to come from head on. It feels like a force, pushing me from the left.

DOUGLAS: That misalignment—can you, as your tears continue, notice the precise direction of the pressure? What is the angle? How many degrees off center is my voice?

B: Twenty.

D: Twenty degrees. Okay, feeling the tension of that twenty degrees, feeling your urge to lower the pressure by reducing the angle of misalignment, wanting so badly to reduce it from twenty to nineteen, to eighteen, all the way down to zero, feeling your tears on your face, needing to reduce the pressure, feeling the pull to *decrease* the angle—go ahead and, counter-intuitively, without moving a muscle, *increase* the angle to twenty-one degrees. Hear my voice coming from twenty-one degrees off center.

Bernice remained silent for a long time. When she next spoke, her tears had stopped and she sounded confused.

B: I don't understand, but the pressure just *diminished*.

D: Yes. Isn't that curious? Funny the way circles work. You can get from your living room to your back yard by going out the back door, or you can head straight out the front door and keep going and going and going and going, and eventually enter it over the back fence. Let's see what happens when you increase the angle to twenty-two degrees.

B: [long pause] More pressure just released.

D: Right. Might as well go to twenty-three degrees.

B: Wow. I don't believe this. The angle just jumped to forty-five degrees. And the pressure keeps getting lower.

D: Great. How much will the angle increase next?

B: It just became ninety degrees. One part is light, the other dark.

The angle continued to increase, from one-hundred-and-twenty to one-hundred-and-eighty degrees and then all the way around to three-hundred-and-sixty. I'm not sure whether Bernice was then comfortably experiencing us back at twenty degrees off kilter, or whether it felt to her that we had achieved perfect alignment (she was, after all, an expert in accounting, not geometry). When she opened her eyes, they once again brimmed with tears, but they were now tears of relief and amazement at how wonderful she felt.

Had I acceded to Bernice's initial, urgent need to physically align her chair with mine, I would have robbed her of the opportunity to discover that she could be relieved of her anxiety without having first to alter her physical environment. Her experiencing freedom in relation to her symptom was facilitated by my protecting my freedom in relation to her.

I nurse the same contrarian thoughts when working with my supervisees. A few years ago, on the first night of a semester-long practicum for new clinicians in our family therapy master's program, one of the students told me how "incredibly nervous" she was at the prospect of seeing her first client, and she pleaded with me to do something—anything!—to take away, or at least significantly reduce, her anxiety. Much to her dismay and frustration, I extolled the virtues of such discomfort, pointing out that her learning would be all the more significant and memorable if her body were to continue working overtime. She escalated her demand that I help her quell her fear, but I stood my ground, telling her that managing anxiety is a wonderful skill to learn as a therapist and that I wouldn't want to undermine her opportunity to take important steps in this direction right at the beginning of her career. I wanted to help her preserve the freedom to feel anxious *and* rise to the occasion of sitting down and chatting with clients (which she did), and I wanted to maintain my freedom not to come to her rescue. By refusing to "save" her, I allowed her to come to the realization that she didn't need me after all—at least not in the way she thought she did.

## Protect Your Session-Organizing Choices

You lose your therapeutic freedom if you let your clients tell you when, how often, or for how long you'll see them, but you also lose it if you allow them to dictate how the sessions themselves should be run. Ever had parents come into a family session, demanding that their teenager sit up and contribute actively to the discussion? The teenager recognizes this as a secret cue to slouch, to look bored or distracted, to drift off for a few minutes, to become fascinated by any handy electronic device, or to reach out for some light reading material. A teenager knows better than anyone how to inform Mom and Dad that nobody can force anybody to do anything. As the parents heat up in response to such challenges to their authority, a naive therapist can easily get caught in the fray, inadvertently causing or contributing to a family confrontation by peppering the teenager with questions, trying to convince or entreat him or her to engage in the conversation, or encouraging the parents to "take control of the situation." Any teenager worthy of the name can stonewall such earnest efforts without breaking a sweat, and his or her parents will come away from such a therapy session still more convinced that their kid is an insolent, intractable loser.

You can avoid such pitfalls by making sure you don't badger or go head-to-head with your clients and by protecting your freedom (and responsibility) to conduct your sessions as you see fit. If a parent (or, for that matter, a teenager) is calling the shots, deciding who should be speaking or who should be silent, then the family might as well have stayed home and saved the cost of your fee. I remember a first session I had with a couple, Wendy and Mark, and their fifteen-year-old son, Joey. The parents were scared and angered by the variety of ways Joey was slipping away from them, and they came to therapy with the goal of getting him straightened out. Joey looked less than pleased about being present, so I treaded carefully, inviting his perspective on what his parents were saying but not asking him for detailed answers. Nevertheless, he *did* talk with me, so I was encouraged about the possibilities, somewhere down the road, of our having some useful conversations.

About halfway through the session, Wendy was giving me some background information she considered pertinent when I noticed, out of the corner of my eye, her husband scowling at her, and her, in response, giving him a quick "go to hell" look. I asked her about what had just passed between them, and she said, "Mark wants me to quit talking so much so that Joey will have to participate more. He thinks that since we're here because of what Joey did, Joey should be answering the questions and explaining himself. Mark doesn't want Joey just sitting there, not saying anything, so he is trying to get me to shut up."

Mark agreed with his wife's interpretation of his scowl: "I just think," he said, "that Joey needs to take some responsibility for his actions." Turning in his chair to face his son, he continued, "Joe, if you have it in your head that you can just sit there and drift off into La-La Land while your mother and I do all the talking, then, let me tell you, you've got another think coming. Big time."

I stepped in at this point. "Mark, you're concerned that if Joe sits quietly enough and I'm not careful, we'll get to the end of the session without his having to have said anything at all."

"You bet."

"Well, I'm very interested in what *each* of you has to say, but I don't have a set format for how I gather information. Today, Wendy may do more of the talking; next time, it might be Joe or you. But I don't equate quality of participation with amount of air time. Listening is also important. Have you noticed how most teenagers have an uncanny ability to appear checked-out while they are taking everything in? And, you know, I never assume that the more talkative a person is, the more likely he or she is to change. So I appreciate your concern, but *I'm* not worried about Joe lacking opinions or lacking the will to let them be known."

My comments were designed to reassure Mark that I was neither incompetent nor oblivious and that he could relax into letting me conduct the session. A few minutes later, Joey interrupted his mother to dispute one of her descriptions, and the issue of his being too quiet disappeared. But I'm not sure he would have spoken up had he thought his father had me in his back pocket.

## Look for Ways that Problems Might Not be Problems After All[16]

A successful stockbroker, impressed by Christopher Reeve's use of hypnosis in his rehabilitative efforts, phoned me to ask if I could give him "motivational hypnotic suggestions." Len told me his "numbers were down," and he was concerned that his fear of failure, which had previously pushed him to work harder, was beginning to have the opposite effect. He wanted me to "put [him] in a trance and tell [his] unconscious" to ignore his fear, to feel less of it, or to be more assertive in spite of it." I explained that I wouldn't presume to tell any part of him what to do, in or out of hypnosis, but I *would* be interested in finding out more about his situation to see if I might be of some kind of assistance.

At the beginning of our first session, Len reiterated his urgent request for help with improved motivation, and once again I stressed my desire to better understand what had been happening with his career and life. If I had agreed simply to do what he asked for, I could only have echoed his own urgings to himself—"Push harder!" "Fight fear!" "Achieve success!" I figured that if such admonishments could be useful, they would have already worked and Len wouldn't have called me in the first place.

I saw Len three times over a two-month period, and we never got around to doing hypnosis. During the first session, I asked how his motivation had been changing, how it now differed from before.[17] He told me that as a young man, he had been a star athlete, and he had learned then that pushing toward success meant pushing away his pain and anxiety. Later, when he went into business, he used the same approach, and it had served him well. He had become wealthy, able to buy the cars, the house, the vacations he desired. In the last several months, though, he had made a number of subtle but noteworthy shifts in how he was responding to his job-, money-, and people-troubles. He had stopped wanting to work as many hours as he had in the past; he didn't really care that he was no longer the top broker in his firm; he had lost interest in buying a new house, despite his wife's demands that they acquire a bigger place; he had recently walked away from buying a new Porsche that he had thought he wanted; and he had finally given up trying to change a desperate brother who had always resisted his efforts to help. Because these shifts were so "out of character" for Len, he was scared that he was losing his edge and that his financial stability and personal security were in danger of crumbling.

Rather than signing on to rectify these unsettling developments, I explored how the changes were, perhaps, a sign of Len's achieving a new level of self-acceptance. Indeed, together we discovered that his "problem with motivation" was, in fact, not a problem at all. Not only did he not need "better" motivation, but also he had, without quite realizing it, begun to find a different and much more satisfying way of relating to risk, fear, and desire—he had learned that letting go is sometimes a more viable option than hanging on. Had we proceeded as he had originally requested, we would have bulldozed over this not-yet-detected change. Instead, in this and the subsequent two sessions, we gave the change a discernible form, which helped to further foster its development.

## Think Systemically

Shirin, a Moslem woman in her mid-thirties, was afraid of her sixteen-year-old son, Ramin, so she brought him to my practicum team at the university, requesting that we teach him anger-management skills. Ramin, predictably furious about being dragged in to see us, sat with his back to the one-way mirror and refused to talk to the therapist. Shirin described the ever-present disdain in Ramin's voice, willful disobedience, two incidents of shoving, and frequent temper outbursts and yelling (including threats of violence).

Since Ramin wanted nothing to do with us, we invited him to sit in the waiting room while we continued the session with his mother. Shirin told us that her son's behaviors had been troubling her for the last year or so but that she'd only become truly frightened over the last several months. The therapist asked about the wedding ring Shirin was wearing on her right hand. She told us that she had moved the ring from her left hand when she left Ramin's father, Akbar, three years earlier. Akbar had wanted to stay together (without, though, giving up his mistress), so she was forced to pursue a divorce unilaterally, finally obtaining it after two years. She continued to wear the ring out of respect for Akbar's parents, who still considered her their daughter-in-law and who refused to take down from their livingroom wall the prominently displayed wedding pictures of Shirin and their son. She continued to attend family functions, and she talked frequently with her ex-mother-in-law on the phone.

Shirin told us that Akbar continued to wait for her to return to the marriage. Ever since she had left him, he had been coming to her house to repair things, demanding in return that she have sex with him. At other times, he would come by for supper and wait around to put his son to bed. After Ramin was asleep, he'd take her into her bedroom. Wanting to keep on good terms for the benefit of her son, she would agree to these encounters, but always, she said, under duress. From time to time they still had sex, despite the fact that Shirin had been dating a man for the last year. She kept expecting Akbar to "get the hint," to realize that she was "through with him," but her having a boyfriend hadn't yet inspired him to get on with his own life. He still seemed to think, she said, that he could demand sex from her whenever he wanted it.

We offered Shirin some hunches about Ramin's behavior. "No one in the family," we said, "seems to acknowledge the legitimacy of the divorce. You've been thinking that your involvement with your boyfriend would be a catalyst for Akbar to let go of you, but it seems, on the contrary, to have convinced him that you are an adulteress. If in his, your son's, and your in-laws' eyes, the marriage is still alive, then they may well be viewing you as no better than a whore. You've been hoping that Ramin would respect you for the strength it took to leave Akbar, but we suspect he disrespects you for cheating on his father. Thus, your efforts to demonstrate your independence are backfiring. Until you can convince everyone that the marriage is truly over, we fear that no amount of anger-management training will make a dent in Ramin's treatment of you."

Shirin looked shocked, but she said she thought we were correct. Ramin, she now recognized, had been unfailingly belligerent around her boyfriend, and his abusive language and behavior had only begun after she'd begun dating. We talked about various ways she could send the message that the divorce was final, including transferring the ring from her right hand to a drawer, giving it back to Akbar (privately or, perhaps even better, publically), telling her ex-inlaws to take down the wedding pictures, making a speech at the next family gathering, refusing to let Akbar in her house, and denying him any further sexual contact.

Shirin returned alone several weeks later and told us that Ramin had stopped threatening, scaring, and shoving her, and that his verbal abuse had stopped. He hadn't transformed into the respectful young man she wished he would be (she still didn't appreciate his tone of voice when he talked to her), but she felt he was now acting like a normal American teenager. He even seemed to be accepting, albeit grudgingly, her boyfriend. Asked her how these changes had come about, Shirin told us that she hadn't wanted to "make a scene" in front of the whole family, so she hadn't made any kind of "announcement," but she *had* taken the ring off, let Akbar know in no uncertain terms that there would be no more sex, and talked to her ex-mother-in-law about removing the pictures. Shirin felt no need to schedule further appointments.

## Offer Alternatives to Using Hypnosis for Remembering Past Abuse

Most people in our culture are drenched with Freudian assumptions about therapy, believing, for example, that therapeutic change requires psychological "healing" and that such healing can only occur once past traumas have been brought into conscious awareness. Insight, according to the logic of the *healing* metaphor, disinfects and sutures the wounds of the past.[18] An unquestioning acceptance of this metaphoric representation is often coupled with the mistaken belief that memories are stored in our brains like files on a computer, simply waiting for the double click of the remembering mouse for them to be opened, nicely preserved, onto the screen of consciousness.

Probably the most troubling request for remembering I've received was from the mother of an adopted five-year-old boy, Cody. Gail wanted to know if I used hypnosis with children and had the equipment to videotape my sessions. When I asked her why, she told me that prior to coming to live with her and her husband the previous year, Cody had been living in a foster home. Cody had had difficulty adjusting to the adoption, so much so that Gail began to suspect that he might have been sexually abused by the father in the foster home. She started asking Cody questions—Did Daddy Jim ever touch your pee pee? Did Daddy Jim ever make you touch him? Where did you touch him? Did he pull his pants down? Did he pull *your* pants down? Where was Mommy Janice when he was touching you?—and his answers were so troubling, they had prompted many follow-up queries.

By the time Gail contacted me, she had, she said, pieced together a fairly complete picture of ongoing abuse. Unfortunately, she went on, Cody wasn't being entirely consistent with his "story," so she wasn't sure which parts were true. Suspecting that he still had feelings for "Daddy Jim" and was secretly trying to protect him, Gail wanted me to "hypnotize Cody and cut through the lies." Having been in psychoanalysis for over ten years, she understood well, she said, that Cody's only hope for psychological health was for someone to help him bring all the details of the abuse to the surface. She had been trying to do this on her own, but when she "realized that Cody was lying," she decided it was time to call in a professional. Gail requested that I use hypnosis to separate truth from fiction, to provide the opportunity for a healthy abreaction, and to record the whole thing on videotape so she could go to the District Attorney and "get the bastard who did this to him locked up." She had called the state's abuse hotline to report what she believed had happened, but to date, as far as she knew, no action had been taken. She hoped the videotape would put a fire under the too-complacent bureaucrats.

Gail had no knowledge of child cognitive development and no awareness of the connection between her questions and Cody's answers. I figured that whatever had or hadn't happened with "Daddy Jim," Cody's descriptions (and possible memories) had to have been significantly shaped by Gail's fearful directive curiosity. What she took to be "lying" could easily be understood as patchwork responses to diverse leading questions. I talked with her for well over an hour, gently explaining how kids think and remember, how questions can shape memories, how kids can best be helped to move beyond traumas, and how attempts to make things better can sometimes make them worse. Apologizing for disappointing her, I told her that hypnosis wouldn't be helpful in illuminating the truth and that bureaucrats in the state's social service agency wouldn't consider a hypnosis-session videotape to be useful evidence for pursuing justice.

By the end of our conversation, Gail had decided (as I hoped she would) that she was more interested in Cody changing some troubling behaviors than in his recalling what had been done to him. I subsequently saw the two of them for a few sessions, interspersed with some appointments involving Gail and her husband. The situation at home became much more manageable and, as far as I could determine, Gail stopped pursuing a remembering-based solution to their struggles.

I believe the most important action I took in this case was to help ease Gail away from her single-minded pursuit of Cody's true memories. Had I simply told her that I refuse to use hypnosis for such purposes, she would have continued, I'm sure, searching for a hypnotherapist. And if she had been unfortunate enough to find someone naive enough to agree to her request, his or her efforts to induce cathartic healing would have continued to subject Cody to the trauma of being sexually abused, regardless of what Daddy Jim had or hadn't done.

If you treat therapy as an occasion for insight-facilitated healing and hypnosis as a device for locating inviolate memories of violation, you're asking for a heap of troubles—therapeutic, ethical, and legal. You'll do better, and so will your clients, if you take the position that remembering and talking about past traumas is *one*, but not the *only* or necessarily the *best*, way to pursue therapeutic change. If you adopt an orientation that's in the ball park of what I'm outlining in this book, you'll be able to respond respectfully to client requests for hypnotic memory enhancement without risking the possibility that you'll inadvertently help create a false memory (see, for example, Bloom, 1994; Crews, 1995; Flemons & Wright, 1999; Johnson, Foley, Suengas, & Raye, 1988; Loftus, 1993; Loftus & Ketcham, 1994; Lynn, Rhue, Myers, & Weekes, 1994; Ofshe & Watters, 1994; Pope, 1996; Reviere, 1996; Schacter, 1996; Spanos, Menary, Gabora, DuBreuil, & Dewhirst, 1991; Spiegel & Scheflin, 1994; Stevenson, 1994; Yapko, 1993, 1994).

When prospective clients ask whether I can assist them in discovering whether they've been abused, I tell them that hypnosis can sometimes help people remember things they've forgotten, but it can also help them remember stuff that never happened. "Trouble is," I explain, "nothing in the experience of the hypnosis-aided remembering itself—neither the vividness of the images, nor the degree of detail—can help you determine whether what seems to be a memory actually is one. There's no internal way of gauging the accuracy of the various parts you're remembering or even the event or events as a whole."[19] This then allows me to segue to a question, as I did with Gail, about what they're hoping to accomplish. If they believe that remembering is a necessary precursor to their dealing with some bothersome symptom, I let them know that other options exist, and I introduce them to alternative ways of thinking about and approaching therapeutic change. If they simply want to satisfy their curiosity, I talk about the painful necessity, at times, of living with uncertainty. Using hypnosis might help them feel more sure about what did or didn't happen, but, I point out, the foundation of their certainty could have significant cracks in it.

# 5

# Your Clients' Relationship with Themselves

I knew that I was a substance whose whole essence or nature is only to think, and which, in order to be, has need of no locus and does not depend on any material thing, in such a way that this self or ego, that is to say, the soul by which I am what I am, is entirely distinct from the body.

—*René Descartes*

William Blake . . . knew that the Poetic Imagination was the only reality. The poets have known these things all through the ages, but the rest of us have gone astray into all sorts of false reifications of the "self" and separations between the "self" and "experience."

—*Gregory Bateson*

It is possible to *become* what you are doing; these times come when pouf!—out you go, and there is only the work. The intensity of your focused concentration and involvement maintains and augments itself, your physical needs decrease, your gaze narrows, your sense of time stops. You feel alert and alive; effort becomes effortless. . . . The noun of self becomes a verb. This flashpoint of creation in the present moment is where work and play merge.

—*Stephen Nachmanovitch*

M istaking his *experience* of conscious awareness for an ontological *truth* about selfhood, Descartes was dead wrong about the mind being "entirely distinct from the body." But if you engage in a little self-reflection, you can understand how he got messed up. Thanks to the separative brilliance of language and consciousness, you, like Descartes, slice and dice with consummate expertise. You see a world full of discrete objects, and your sense of self is rife with rifts. This Cartesian mode of understanding works pretty well for conducting experiments, building houses, or locating distant nebulae, but it's horribly suited to understanding or solving problems of the heart-and-mind—to finding and repairing the tears in the fabric of our relationships.

When you think to yourself, "*my* legs hurt," or "I *have* an idea," or "*my* depression is getting to me," you are drawing a line that separates your sensations, thoughts, and emotions from the "self" who "owns" or "has" them. The line is imaginary, a figment of your Cartesian imagination, but this doesn't prevent you from making assumptions and taking action as if the line were real. In Chapter 1, I talked about the homuncular self, the *i,* that results from such line drawing. Your *i*—that little, self-proclaimed CEO of you—considers itself the owner and controller of your experience. Believing its own propaganda, it assumes that it really is a distinct entity, capable of keeping the rest of you in check, and that the way to do this is to control or negate (disown) any sensation, thought, or emotion that it deems unsavory. Trouble is, given the associational foundation of mind, neither strategy can work, at least for any length of time. Dissociative efforts necessarily create separated connections: pain that won't budge, thoughts that won't stop racing, emotions that won't lighten. This is where hypnosis comes into the picture.

Remember what I told you in Chapter 1 about the words *trance* and *transit* sharing a common Latin root? Both have to do with movement, with crossing over something (*trans,* across + *ire,* to go). I find *trance* a useful term for referring to the special relationship people develop with themselves when the boundary between mind and body is crossed over—the boundary that, during times of normal conscious dissociation, separates the *i* from the rest of the self. Curious things happen to your sense of self when you start crossing the boundaries that define who and what you are, as well as where "you" begin and end. Let me give you few diverse examples.

Growing up in Canada, I, like many English speakers in my country, devoted a fair bit of time to figuring out what it means to be Canadian. My working definition depended much on two negations: I wasn't quite British (despite my English and Scottish heritage, my knowing all the words to "God Save the Queen," and the presence of the Queen's visage on our currency), and I sure as hell wasn't American (despite—or, more likely, because of—being enthralled by, inundated with, and afraid of American culture and politics).

When I first traveled as a teenager to England in 1972, I encountered many people who let me know that my hailing from one of "the colonies" guaranteed my not-British identity. I encountered the opposite attitude when I met Americans, either in my or their country. They didn't care much where I was born, and they didn't get the "Canadian thing." Sure, I pronounced a few words in an amusing way, but other than that, they didn't know what all the fuss was about. Why bother distinguishing between us?—American? Canadian? What did it matter? Well, it mattered to *me,* and, in response to their ignorance of what I considered my national uniqueness, I, like many Canadians, redoubled my efforts to assert my not-Americanness.

The Brits erected a boundary that kept me an outsider; the Yanks ignored a boundary that I deemed essential. So what or who was I? A British wannabe and an American don't-wannabe. My identity as a Canadian depended entirely on the inscribing of boundaries—either by others or myself.

Years later, I moved to the States, developed close friendships with many Americans, married my American wife, Shelley, and, with her, produced Eric and Jenna, our two American/Canadian children. Not wanting to exclude myself from Americans I care about, and no longer caring about British exclusivity, I lost a lot of my nationalist zeal, and, with it, my means of defining myself as a Canadian. As my boundary-marking changed, so did my sense of identity.

If you put me in conversation with an American who is clueless about Canada and its relationship to the States, my nationalist boundaries will likely appear out of nowhere. But most of the time, my Canadian identity isn't nudged into prominence.

Boundaries configure your identity internationally, but also inter- and intrapersonally. When differences stop making a difference, when boundaries become irrelevant, the distinctiveness of the "thing" they create disappears. Remember how, in Chapter 1, I talked about the dissolution of the sense of self that happens when you're singing in a choir? When you and those around you are all producing the same note, the sound frequency on both sides of your ear drum is the same, so the boundary separating inside and outside disappears and, with it, your sense of being an isolated self. Something similar, if less dramatic, happens at mealtime. If your partner eats garlic and you don't, you will later smell the result of your different meals; however, if you both eat garlic, *neither* of you will smell it. Like the same term appearing on both sides of an equation,

$$6y(2) = 4x(3)$$
$$12y = 12x$$
$$y = x$$

the smell is canceled out. Where there's no difference, there's no boundary, and where there's no boundary, there's no perception.

The experience of hypnosis similarly depends on the de-demarcating of a boundary, in this case, the intrapersonal boundary that defines ordinary consciousness. When you are in trance, your *i* stops distinguishing itself as "the thinker," separate from your thoughts; as "the perceiver," separate from your perceptions; as "the feeler," separate from your emotions. During hypnosis, your conscious awareness isn't marking itself as distinct, claiming credit and authority for all your cognitioning and emotioning; instead, you experience the mindfulness of your body and the embodiment of your mind. This is the special relationship of hypnosis, or better, as I suggested in Chapter 1, of *concordance*—a relationship where you are of one mind-and-heart with yourself. Such concordance is an instance of metaphoric knowing, an experience, for the duration of the trance, of the identity of mind and body. As in the equation above, where y = x, the distinction between your *i* and the rest of you becomes, for the period of your being in concordance with yourself, irrelevant.

When you're in trance, you don't stop distinguishing altogether—you don't lose, for example, your ability to understand language or to think or perceive. But rather than your having the sense, as you usually do, that you are (that is, that your *i* is) doing your thinking from some removed vantage, you experience yourself *inside* your thinking, feeling, sensing, moving. No longer separate from these mindful processes, you lose the sense that your *i* is in control; however, as I point out to my clients, this isn't a real loss, because "you" weren't in control in the first place (see Bateson, 2000). Caught up in the Cartesian delusions of everyday consciousness, "you" just thought you were. Anytime you have a focused connection with something and/or someone, your conscious habit of distinguishing stops folding back on itself, stops isolating your *i* as an object (or, more accurately, as a subject) that takes all the credit for any and all mindful activity.[1]

Concordance creates the conditions for your mindful body and embodied mind to experience a free play of ideas, images, and feelings—a relational freedom that would be difficult, if not impossible, to introduce within the dissociative context of conscious thought. Dissociations are common within hypnotic experiencing, but they are *associated* dissociations—gaps of insignificance (see Chapter 1) or connected separations that can only arise within the associative context of one-mindedness. If you were to enter a hypnotic relationship with me, you might feel numb or find yourself floating, far away from your body or my voice; you might get so involved in an image or unfolding narrative that you would lose track of your surroundings and of time, later forgetting what happened; or your body or a sensation might seem like it has a mind of its own, capable of moving or changing without your *i* being in charge of it. Within this changed relationship with yourself, you could entertain and experience a changed relationship with your problem (see Chapter 6), which is the point at which hypnosis becomes hypnotherapy.

In Chapter 4, I explained the importance of your helping your clients become of one mind with you. This is essential if you are to facilitate their becoming of one mind with themselves and if you are, together, to make therapeutic use of their intrapersonal concordance. In this chapter, I use a detailed transcript of a hypnotherapy session to clarify and illustrate how this can happen. The session is the fourth of five I had with Anna, a single mother experiencing pain in the joints of her fingers, hands, and hips. Her joints had been irritating her for several years, affecting her sleep, concentration, and ability to work, and they sometimes prevented her from gripping things with her hands. For about six weeks before our first appointment, every joint in her body, except her elbows, had been hurting with a "swollen, achy, burny feeling." Whenever the pain worsened, Anna worried about becoming debilitated, which seemed to further exacerbate the symptoms. Steroid injections had provided only shortterm relief, and Anna's digestive system couldn't handle the nonsteroidal anti-inflammatories her doctor prescribed.

Between the third and fourth session, Anna's pain had lessened for a few days, and she had begun to hope that the hypnosis might be capable of helping her. She figured she had "over done it," though. Feeling better, she had gone back to the gym and had carried heavy packages from the grocery store "like a normal person," resulting in a flare-up. In earlier sessions, I had offered some guidance for how Anna could try self-hypnosis at home, so at the beginning of our appointment, I followed up with how it had been working. She told me that she had had trouble staying with it long enough to "wind her mind down." Just like when she used to try to meditate, her mind wouldn't empty, but rather wandered as she thought of all the things she had to do.

I told her that self-hypnosis is not about "trying to get into trance by emptying your mind" or about "trying to get some place *other* than where you are." I wondered whether she'd been telling herself, "Here I am, and I need to be over *there* in order to be in a trance, but I can't get over there because of something going on here (I'm too wired, too distracted, too wound up)." She agreed that she been distracted and irritated by her conscious thinking, so I explained that instead of asking, "What can I do to get my mind empty?" she might just set aside the time for hypnosis and figure out where she *was* instead of where she had to *get to,* because "the place *to get* really is where you *are.*"

Anna thought this sounded a lot like daydreaming—an activity that had always come naturally and easily to her. I agreed that there were many similarities, including inner absorption. Anna had been working hard *not* to daydream, as she had thought it would screw up the hypnosis. On the contrary, I said, you can use the one to make the other possible.

DOUGLAS: You could start a daydream.
ANNA: [scratches chin, smiles] Is anyone reading my mind? [laughs]
D: What's nice about daydreams is that they're perfectly private.

If Anna was worried that being of one mind with me wouldn't be safe, that I'd somehow have too much access to her private thoughts, she'd need to maintain a boundary between us. By reassuring her that I couldn't trespass, I offered her the possibility of relaxing into the relationship, of venturing concordance.

A: I know. [pause] Daydreams. Starting one on purpose—I've never ever done in my life.
D: Really?
A: I just, there's a *thought,* and I like the *thought,* so I stay with the *thought* and it develops into a story.
D: Huh. How often does that happen?
A: I don't know, it depends on how busy I am or if I have time for those things. Of course I had them a lot when I was little. [nods] In Latin classes and things like that.
D: You can't *make* it happen but you can just plant a seed?
A: No, what happens is a thought comes into my head and if I have time to play with it and develop it, if I have energy and time, desire to play with it and develop it, then it *will* become a daydream. If I don't have time, then it doesn't get developed, certainly not for any length of time.
D: If you *take* the time to develop it nicely, how long does it last? [she looks up to the ceiling] The whole daydream?
A: [looks at me] I don't know, I've never paid attention, it's so natural, it's so, I'm sure you do it, too. It's just so automatic, I guess I never paid attention to, "Gee, I just whiled away an hour on this," because I can do things while I'm daydreaming, too. I mean, I can go

through *motions* of doing things. I couldn't sit down and do *bills* or
anything. I don't know, I guess I never really made any distinctions
with it. It's just part of my life.

D: Well, it's interesting. Perhaps what you've been trying to do is to
think that you need to do something *other* than daydreaming.

If, to experience hypnosis, she had to work at not daydreaming, she'd
be sunk. Attempting to negate thoughts, images, and stories as they
developed would only reinforce the boundary between them and the
*i* that was trying to control them. By accepting—indeed, inviting—
daydreams, her *i* and her thought processes could be of one mind, and
the distinction between them could become indistinct.

A: Yeah, maybe. That may be. Oh, I'm sure I could daydream. But
see, that's what I thought was happening, that I was beginning to
daydream when I was trying to go into a trance and be specific
about something, that my mind would wander into daydreams
and that, in fact, was disturbing my trance.

D: Oh, okay. Well then, that's

A: That's wrong, huh?

D: that's my, that's my misdirection for you if you were left with that
impression.

I always take responsibility for my clients' misunderstandings and
confusions. I'd rather them blame me than themselves.

D: What you want to do with the trance is, you set up a *possibility,* not
an agenda. So you'd set up a possibility—"I wonder," for example,
you could ask yourself a question, "I wonder how my unconscious,
or my daydreaming, will continue to help me feel healthier?"—and
something as general and vague as that. And then you leave it up to
your unconscious—you leave it up to the part that you have no
control over—to decide what on earth it wants to daydream.

Milton Erickson pointed out that self-hypnosis often goes awry
when you start trying to give yourself suggestions. He recommended
asking yourself a question (such as the one I was suggesting that

Anna pose) at the beginning of your time with yourself, and then sitting back and waiting to see what happens. The approach is a good one because it helps you avoid reintroducing the Cartesian boundary between the part of you that's supposedly thinking up and delivering the suggestions (your *i*) and the part that is supposed to be listening and responding to them.

I mentioned her "unconscious" here, and I did so again a few more times throughout the session, but I'm not terribly enamored of the notion. Making reference to your clients' unconscious can allow you to talk about the parts of their knowing and experience that lie outside their conscious scrutiny, and this can help engender relational freedom between them and their problems, but I get edgy when people reify the unconscious, turning it into a concrete entity. I have no trouble talking about your conscious awareness or your *i* as a "thing" because that's how you experience it, or, more accurately, that's how it experiences itself. As I said in Chapter 1, your *i* is a "thing-thinker," a "thingker." But unconscious processes aren't *object*-oriented—they're *relationship*-oriented.

You perceive by drawing distinctions (Bateson, 2000), discriminating objects by separating them from their surroundings. You don't perceive relationships unless you isolate them (as things), so most of the time, the associational processes of mind that undergird and contextualize your consciousness go, by definition, unnoticed. Put differently, your unconscious only becomes a thing when you draw conscious attention to it. Left to its own devices, it isn't an "it."

I generally prefer, then, to talk to clients about their body-knowledge rather than about their "unconscious." This avoids the reification problem, and we never get sidetracked by questions about Freud. Nevertheless, invoking Anna's unconscious here helped me to suggest that Anna didn't need to set part of herself off as the CEO of her experience, that her *i* didn't need to control or assume a "meta" position as the interpreter of what happened.

D: And to not worry about having to interpret it, or make sense of it, that it's "on task,"
A: Uh huh.

D: but that you allow it to develop on its own. And then the daydream
   can be helpful for reasons and in ways that you don't understand,
   and that you might not recognize, even if you were to follow the
   daydream closely and scrutinize it, take notes, that it would still be
   doing what it's doing quite apart from your conscious scrutiny.

Her scrutinizing, she had said earlier, was getting in the way of her
developing a trance, but if she had tried to stop it—tried to control
her controlling—she would have only further sliced her sense of herself, further demarcating the division between her *i* and her experience. I thus welcomed the scrutiny and indicated its limitations,
opening the possibility that Anna wouldn't have to *bother* keeping
track of what was happening. For the scrutinizing to become a non-
issue, it needed to become unnecessary.

A: Maybe I haven't even done enough daydreaming lately, 'cause I've
   been too busy. That could be a problem in my life, [laughing] 'cause
   it's really, I loved it—my daydreams—I've always, . . . it just,
   I'm, when it starts to happen I may notice it more and just let it
   happen.
D: Well, why don't you let it happen right now? [pause while she
   smiles] 'Cause I'm going to talk, [she nods] but this is not like
   paying bills.

I used "let it happen" to segue from a *discussion* about doing something different with her daydreaming at home to an *invitation* that
she do something different with it in the moment. She had said earlier that she couldn't daydream *and* do bills, but why not daydream
*and* experience hypnosis? That way, what had been an impediment to
trance could become a conduit.

A: This is not like paying bills. [laughs as she repositions herself on
   the couch] Good. There's nothing worse than paying bills.
D: So, you don't need to listen to me.
A: So, I don't need to listen to you. I can tune you out.
D: You can tune me out and you get into your best dream time that
   you can manage. [she looks up, then nods] Okay. Now you don't
   *have* to tune me out, however.

If you have a background in hypnosis, you might well be saying to yourself at this point, "Okay, there he goes, he's started the induction." The word *induce* comes from the Latin *inducere,* to lead into, to introduce. I don't think of inductions as a separate stage in the hypnotic process, and I dislike the commonly held assumption that in inducing hypnosis, the therapist is doing something *to* his or her clients. My job, as I see it, is to *invite, facilitate, and maintain concordance* between me and my clients and between them and themselves.

A:  [overlapping] I don't have to tune you out. Okay.

If she didn't have to listen to me and didn't have to *not* listen to me, then she'd have no need to enter into a self-other relationship with herself (where her *i* was trying to stop whatever it determined she was doing wrong). Instead, she could enter into a win-win concordance with herself, as well as with me.[2]

D:  And what you might do is imagine yourself then at home now with yourself propped up in your bed and with a special pillowcase or the special cover, or the special animal, or whatever dream [pause, then she engages my eyes] marker you're going to use.

With the pause between "dream" and "marker," I began the shift in the pacing of my words, slowing down and speaking in time with Anna's breathing. By linking the rhythm of my speech with the rhythm of her body, I was, as most hypnotists do, conspiring (from the Latin *con,* together + *spirare,* breathe: to breathe together) to ensure that our concordance was *embodied.*[3]

My mentioning the special pillowcase, cover, and animal related back to some ideas I had offered earlier in the session (prior to where the transcript starts) about ways she could, in her very small living space, contextually mark off space and time for self-hypnosis.

D:  This is dream time. It might be just something that, something small that you hold in your hand, or it simply could be something that you wear but that [pause as she stretches the fingers of her right hand and then makes a fist] you hold tightly to the necessity to be able to go down,

My "hold tightly" further connected my words and her body movement.

D:  or go into a trance [she opens her fingers, resting her right hand on
     her leg] by going into a dream. And you don't need an agenda and
     you don't need to try hard, and your mind wandering often is a nice
     way to start a daydream, isn't it?
A:  [nods] Hmm hmm.
D:  And so it's really not, [she clears her throat] there's not a right way
     to get there. You can meander your way in if meandering is your
     chosen way of getting absorbed in your own experience. [pause
     while she nods slightly and then adjusts her position]

Meandering wouldn't be efficient, obviously, for her getting to some
distant goal, but hypnosis is never out there, apart; rather, it is in the
process of proceeding. By suggesting that she could meander, I was
inviting her to let go of her goal-directed thinking, of her purposefully trying to create a hypnotic relationship with herself.

D:  So you could imagine that you're home [she nods very slightly] and
     that you're finding that way to absorb, and as you move further into
     the dream you can just position yourself, [I uncross and recross my
     legs] whatever is most comfortable for you. [she scratches her face
     with her right hand]

If she were to able to imagine herself at home, then she'd already be
developing a connected separation between her physical and imagined locations. Such associated dissociations characterize all hypnotic
phenomena.

D:  Though here you have the benefit of my voice, but as I said, you
     can choose to tune that out if it's getting in the way [she nods
     slightly] of your developing a good dream. That ability as a young
     girl to have a thought, a good thought that somehow grabs you,

She had told me that she developed her daydreaming skill as a young
girl. My comment referenced that history, but it also gently suggested another connected separation: age regression. By using the

present-tense *grabs,* rather than the past-tense *grabbed,* I was offering the possibility that she could experience herself *in the present* as a young girl.

D: and to be able to play with it [she is blinking occasionally, and her eyes remain focused on mine] until it develops into a story.

As Sandra Roscoe pointed out (Roscoe, 1996), describing a thought in terms of its ability to *grab* and to be *played with* imbues mind with body-like physicality, thereby further bridging the mind-body gap of ordinary consciousness. The process of a thought turning into a story was something Anna had discussed earlier in the session.

D: You can have that thought now, if you haven't already got one [pause] and begin even perhaps out of your conscious awareness to develop it. [her blinking slows] The nice thing about having a daydream and the nice thing about going into trance is that your conscious mind doesn't need to be involved, and it can *try* to be involved and you can let it help if it really wants to, I guess. You can humor it.

Language and consciousness deliver us a dissociated sense of ourselves. When you say, "I'm trying not to go back for seconds" or "I couldn't help myself—my temper got the best of me," you experience yourself as divided. Your *i* distinguishes itself from, and attempts to control, such "irrational" pulls and pushes. Grappling with the rest of you, it tries—usually not successfully and often with some degree of exasperation—to get your thoughts, habits, desires, sensations, and emotions to do its bidding, to bend to its disjunctive will.

By offering the idea that Anna could "humor" her conscious mind, I was turning the presumptions of her *i* upside down, implying that her sense of self could extend beyond the boundaries of her conscious awareness. I was also offering her a connective strategy for dealing with its separatist proclivities. Rather than trying to pull away from or control her *i,* she could simply let it be, recognizing that its contributions were not significant.

D: But knowing that what really matters is that you find your way in to where you are now, so if you have your mind [her right fingertips

gently touch her left ones] winding up and racing that you then just
race with it and *follow alongside it* and listen for a while to the
racing.

I again offered body-based descriptions of her mind; later, you will
see that I also did the reverse, attributing mind-like abilities to various parts of her body (Roscoe, 1996).

D:  [her blinking slows further] And you might even see if you can
    speed it up just a bit more so that it's racing at just the right speed.

If she were to try to slow down or stop her thoughts, Anna would be
at odds with them, thereby further reinforcing the Cartesian division
between her *i* and the rest of herself, and nailing the coffin on her
intrapersonal concordance. Exercising my contrarian thinking (see
Chapter 4), I encouraged her, instead, to connect with the racing,
which, of course, was a way for her to connect with herself, allowing
the distinction between her *i* and her thoughts to become indistinct.

D:  [more quickly] And you know when you drive quickly in a nice car
    that you can be going very fast and it begins to feel like you're
    going [softly and slowly] quite slow-ly. [pause] And so as you get in
    *time* with the racing, the car seems to *ssslowww* [she blinks and
    swallows] way down.

Think of the last time you were leaning forward, skiing at break-
neck speed down a mountain or riding your bicycle with the wind at
your back. As long as you weren't afraid of crashing, you felt like you
were gliding effortlessly, right? When your awareness is in sync with
your movement, your pace seems nice and slow. The same thing happens when your *i* is keeping up with the movement of your *thoughts*.
When it and they are of one mind, the racing-out-of-control sensation disappears.

D:  It's only when you're accelerating and you're a little bit behind
    where the car is that you can feel that pull, but once you're there and
    the two of you, the car and you, are at full speed, it's then possible for
    you to just [softly] calmly steer your way, and that's a good time

often to daydream as well. You can attend to what you need to be safe and then [pause as she blinks and looks away from my eyes] free up yourself [pause] to absorb yourself in your experience. Now that may not be a good time for you [she reengages my eyes] and certainly it matters for you to find the time that's best for you, but the principle [her right hand clasps her left wrist and both hands move closer to her waist, where they remain motionless for the next several minutes] is the same. That you can carry on with what you're doing *now* and race and consider everything that's going on in your head [pause] right [pause] now. You could itemize them all.

I was making a brief, oblique reference back to the bill paying.

D:  You could itemize them backwards. [she again looks away from eyes and continues to rest her gaze down to the left of me]

More contrarian thinking.

D:  You could follow them as they make their course and all of the jumps and leaps and wondering where you're going to go next.

Notice my continued use of body-based metaphors for describing the movement of her thoughts. My suggestion that she be playful, rather than directive, with her thinking was designed to further her being of one mind with it.

D:  And in the midst of all that hustle and bustle and rustle, allow that storyline to develop [pause] itself. And so there can be at least three things going on simultaneously. You can be listening or not listening to my voice, [pause] you can be racing with your *conscious* mind, or it might be racing with questions about what I'm saying, or it could be about work or about plans or about Thomas [her son] or about your fingers, but it could be any number of things.

I, too, wanted to keep up with her racing, providing her with lots of possibilities for what she could think about.

D:  And then the storyline, all on *its* own, developing [pause] nicely

Most novelists will tell you that they have little, if any, control over the stories they create. When their writing is going well, they feel as if the story is inventing itself or as if the characters have taken over and are calling all the shots. We can orient ourselves so as to *facilitate* such invention (< Latin *in,* in + *venere,* to come: to come into), but we can't steer it directly.

Anna knew well how to allow the storyline to develop on its own, how to let go of any attempt to consciously control it. A daydream is an experience of relational freedom, made possible by the connected separation between the dreamer and the dream. I figured that this particular freedom could help usher in other nonvolitional (i.e., hypnotic) changes in her experience.

D:  and privately, [softly] *always privately.*

I wanted to make sure that she felt safe, so I reiterated my assurance that our concordance wouldn't threaten her privacy. The safer she felt, the more she could relax into a connected relationship with me and with herself.

D:  And that experience can be [her blinking slows] then threefold at
    least. But then there is the question of what is the relationship
    between [pause, then her eyes close for a moment] the first [pause]
    conscious thought [she meets my gaze again] you have and the
    second one in order how did you make that leap?

Asking about the *relationships between* her thoughts was a way of inviting her to move from her conscious thingking into the associational, interstitial thinking characteristic of hypnosis.

D:  [her eyelids flutter] And then the relationship between these two
    thoughts and the storyline developing [she looks down to my right] all
    on its own. And whatever those have to do with each other, and then
    the relationship between the two conscious or three conscious thoughts,
    one after the other, the relationship between them and the developing
    narrative of the [her eyes close and stay closed for the rest of the session]
    storyline, and then that with my voice and what I'm saying, that's
    right. And it may even be a relationship of no relationship.

I was covering all possibilities with this last comment, in case she was saying to herself, "Relationship? What relationship?" Later, I invited her into the relationships between different parts of her body.

D:  One can continue [I speak over to her right] all on its own over there, and the other can continue [I speak over to her left] all on its own over there, and the third can continue [I speak directly to her] on over here, [softly] all on its own.

By using the direction of my voice to assign a particular location in space for each of the three kinds of experiences, I was indirectly suggesting that they could be teased apart. I located the third one—developing a storyline—right in front of her, directly between the two of us. I wanted to link it to our concordance.

D:  And how nice that you've known ever since you were a little girl how to go [softly] into this special state where you find *you*. [pause]

Just because I don't conceptualize hypnosis as a special state (see Chapter 1) doesn't mean my clients don't *experience* it as one.

D:  And allow your imagination to run, [pause] and jump, [pause] and tumble, [her left index and middle fingers twitch] that's right, [she momentarily lifts all her left fingers] and play.

My body-based descriptions of thought processes had moved beyond the notion of "racing thoughts" to evoking the freedoms of childhood games, thus furthering the evocation of an age regression. I returned to this later in the session.

Sometimes when clients tell me that their racing thoughts are precluding their experiencing hypnosis, I talk to them about how wolf packs work. "Wolves need to patrol the perimeter of their territory," I say, "but if all of them were to do this all the time, none of them would get a chance to rest. So they take turns. Part of the pack keeps moving, always moving, along the edge of their territory, making sure everything is safe and secure, while the rest are able, in the center, to relax deeply. That continual prowling, that continual circling along the territorial edge is essential for the well-being of the pack as a whole, allowing them to relax into the security of feeling protected. So you could always adopt the wisdom of the wolves, allowing part of you to continue prowling, continue circling around, continue allowing the rest of you to rest, the rest of you to let go into the knowledge that you are being kept safe by that loping, that circling, that scrutiny of the edge, the edge of trance." And so on.

D: That's right. And how different your experience becomes once you begin [pause] running, [pause] allowing your imagination to turn somersaults [pause] to twirl, [pause as people are walking down the hall outside the room, talking and closing doors] and be just as aware of whatever happens outside of here as you need be, but let it . . . just . . . pass . . . by.

The people walking down the hall were so loud, I figured I'd best incorporate them into my talk. Had Anna at the time seemed more fully absorbed in our relationship and her own experience, I probably wouldn't have bothered mentioning the noise they were making. But since she wasn't, I was happy for the opportunity to differentiate the people *outside* the room from the two of us *inside* it. With Anna's attention focused on the boundary separating her and I from the outsiders, it would less likely be drawn to distinguishing herself from me or from other parts of her experience. The interruption could thus help her and my, as well as her own, concordance.

D: And how nice to let that dream develop and enter into dream time. The nice thing about dreams, of course, is how real they can become, that inside of the dream, you're not even, aware that it isn't a dream,

This sense of experiential reality is true not only of dreams, but also of hypnosis.

D: and that the movement through [pause] terrain, encountering people [she coughs] can continue as you clear the way for the story to develop. [pause]

My "clear the way," in response to her cough, turned an interruption into a sound effect in support of a change in awareness.

D: And each time that you've been here the experience has been
slightly different, and you might indeed find *this* experience
developing in the same way as last time, and yet different in some
small or sig*nificant* way. [fingers on both her hands begin to move;
the right hand closes into a loose fist, opens, and then closes again]
That's right. How nice it is to feel your hands feeling different
again, and I wonder how the daydream [pause] could incorporate
that [pause while her right hand lightly rubs her right shoulder
before returning to her lap] and always move to get comfortable
[pause while she entwines her fingers] and let the fingers talk to one
another [long pause] and you can always count [pause] on your
fingers. [pause while her fingertips move slightly]

The pun about her counting on her fingers made another implicit reference to childhood activities (children use their fingers for counting),
and it sprinkled in the notion that Anna, despite feeling betrayed by
her body, could begin to trust it, to count on it.

Some therapy models, such as Alcoholics Anonymous, rely on
teaching clients how they can never trust themselves. Whenever possible, I head in the opposite direction, encouraging people to trust
their guts, their hope, their fingers, their voices, their reservations,
*and* their negative experiences.

To further (and to indirectly) enliven the "counting on/trusting"
pun, I began counting from one to seven, embedding the numbers
into the flow of my descriptions (I'll point them out to you in square
brackets).

D: One [1] way to do that is to recognize that you have two [2] hands
[long pause] and yet when they're entwined, [her fingertips
continue to move; her head inclines slightly forward] it's almost
perhaps as if there's a third [3], that is, a combination of the two.
[long pause] And what can that third hand reach out and do [her
thumbs straighten and their tips momentarily push against each
other, then she pauses] now . . . *for* [4] . . . you. [she takes a deep,
long breath]

A third hand, one that arose from the combination of the other two,
would, I reasoned, be pain free.

D:  And you don't need to try to do anything at all. In fact, you could
even try *trying* and realize that that's not part of your experience of
going even deeper down into trance. [pause]

Offering her the option of "trying to try" was intended to free her
up from trying to *not try*. If she *were* to try to try and discover that
it did indeed get in the way of her concordance with herself, then
the experience would further her concordance with me (because I
predicted its happening). If she decided just not to bother trying
to try, then she wouldn't be attempting to control her experience,
which would help facilitate her connection with herself. A win-win
situation.

Your clients must *slip* into the metaphoric experience of hypnosis.
If they try to help you create their concordance with themselves, their
efforts will maintain the differences between you, as well as the
mind-body split within themselves. To invite them out of their
everyday disembodiment—as a conscious *i* separate from their
body—you need to find a way to free them from the responsibility for
making trance happen. Released to float within, rather than having
to steer, the process, they can more easily become of one mind with
you and themselves.

D:  There was a movie once, "Five [5] Easy Pieces,"

I was only guessing that she'd know this reference to a film in which
Jack Nicholson plays a pianist. But even if the oblique association
"easy piece on the piano = easy (i.e., flexible) finger movement"
went over her head (over her fingers?), my mentioning the title allowed me to say the number *five* and to contrast "trying" with "easy."

D:  and there's nothing easier than just letting yourself move [pause]
where you are and find yourself there, find yourself in your hands,
allow your hands to continue to elaborate their *own* thinking, their
*own* knowing, because they know how to do so much on their own.

I had earlier offered numerous body-based descriptions of her thinking; here, I balanced this with mindful descriptions of her body and
the idea of her *i* relaxing its controlling grip on her hands.

D:  How nice to listen to them tell a story [long pause] because in a
    way really that is what happens is it not when you go down into a
    daydream, that you allow your *body* to tell you a story, one that
    you don't plan out but that gets told. [she takes a deep long
    breath]

This notion of her hands having a story to tell arose from her earlier
description of how her daydreams typically developed. A spontaneous story would be one with relational freedom, one with which
she could have a connected separation.

D:  Of course, if you were to multiply the number of hands you *do* have
    [2] by the number of hands that are created by that combination
    [3], [her left index finger lifts momentarily] that is one less than the
    seven [7] Samurai that it took to [various fingers move slightly]
    make such a difference in that town [$2 \times 3 = 6$]. [long pause,
    during which her right fingers disengage from the left ones, she
    reaches up and lightly rubs the corner of her right eye, and then her
    right hand rests on her left wrist]

Another film reference—this one to Kurosawa Akira's "The Seven
Samurai." I wish I could tell you that I knew Anna was a film buff,
but I can't because I didn't. I don't know if the film titles meant anything to her.

D:  Your hands know so much about how to bring relief. [she shifts her
    position slightly]

I was ostensibly talking about her hands' ability to relieve itches (see
below), but I also intended the remark as an introduction to the idea
that her hands, the source of so much pain, could bring a more profound kind of relief—relief from pain.

D:  Without thinking, they can scratch [pause while her left fingers
    flex] and move [her left hand makes a loose fist] and hold. And [her
    left fingers straighten] I wonder what they would like to hold onto,
    what they would like to continue to hold onto and never let go of.
    [pause]

My "scratch and move" described her body movement; the phrase "hold onto" gave metaphorical significance to her fist-making, further connecting her body, my words, and her mind. Her emphasis had been on her hands getting rid of the pain. I, in my contrarian fashion, wanted to establish the presumption that they had something to hold onto.

D:  What really matters to them to hold onto *tightly,* and never let go of, [her right fingers move slightly] and before you move deeper into trance, you might find yourself asking them to tell *you* what *they hold dear.* [long pause while her lips move and she swallows]

I was continuing to distinguish Anna's sense of self from her body, but the division wasn't between a thinking *i* and a non-thinking body. In floating the possibility for her and her hands to talk with each other, I was proposing that she and they could, via a thought-full conversation, become of one mind. Anna had told me at the beginning of the session that she had been trying to deal with the pain by ignoring it, by pushing it away. I was offering, instead, a connective strategy. Hands are for holding. What's important for them to hold onto?

D:  Because just like you, they want to take their time developing their own understanding [long pause as her right arm and hand move slightly] and you can consciously check them out for the changes that are going on there, but, they have their own *knowing* that's much deeper than that, and what do *they* wish to hold onto?

My comment was intended as a kind of insurance policy. Given the amount of moment-to-moment scrutiny of her joints she'd been engaging in over the last several weeks, I wanted to cover the possibility of her looking for changes and not noticing any. If this were to happen, then instead of immediately discounting our work together, she might conclude that she simply wasn't able to consciously monitor it. I was hoping to introduce a connected separation between her expectations and the changes her body could undergo.

D:  And allow them to tell a story to each other about that. I don't know—if they were to have a conversation, who would be the one to

lead it? [she sits still, then her fingers entwine for a moment
before she reaches up to rub the corner of her right eye; her right
hand then returns to her lap and her fingers entwine] Imagine for
a moment that your right hand is your left, your left, your right
[pause] so that the signals that your right hand are sending to
your left brain become the signals that your left hand would be
sending your right brain if your, [her hands return to her lap, each
lightly clasping the other; her head remains on the back of the
couch] your left hand were your right hand sending signals to your
left brain. And so allow your right index finger to become your
left index finger. [pause] And you know [the tips of her index
fingers touch] . . . [long pause] how your hands can cradle each
other and take care of each other. [long pause] Then allow that
dream or that story to begin to unfold. [long pause; her fingers
remain entwined as her hands move closer to her waist] And what
do your hands have to contribute to that story? [her body remains
very still during a very long pause]

If right becomes left and left right, then the distinction between
them stops mattering. If she could lose track of which hand was
which, I reasoned, then this might change the perception of pain associated with a particular joint on a particular hand.

D:  And you needn't *try* [pause] anything, you needn't try [her right
hand scratches right temple] to go into a trance. But you might
wonder where the next itch will be, anticipate it, and wonder what
your mind and your hand is thinking as it travels up to relieve it.
[her fingers move slightly before coming still again, then a long
pause] In what way will it next bring you relief [pause] and how
will it make the trip? Will it make it slowly or quickly?

As you can see from reading the body-movement descriptions in
the transcript, Anna's hands moved a lot, often in a way that I interpreted at the time as indicative of her not being in concordance with
herself. I thus continued to sprinkle in comments intended to connect both of us to these movements. Sometimes I do this through
puns. I'll suggest to people who continue to scratch themselves that
they begin to pay attention to that itch, that itch within them for

something to be different. And when stomachs growl, I might throw in a reference to the "rumblings of change," and so on.

D:  I knew a man once who did his dissertation on the fact that we are all elegant. He did that by photographing people lifting glasses of water of various weights, and he filmed it and was able to prove that we adjust the speed at which we lift and the muscles used, depending on perceived weight, and so just before your next relief and itch, you might want to just wait [pause] but a moment [pause] [her fingers move a little] in order to consider the trajectory. And how does your hand know where to *find it?* [very long pause] How does it make *that* movement, [softly] *that one?* [her hands unclasp] Your conscious mind can wonder about what you're feeling there in your hands. [pause, then her fingertips push against each other] Test it like a good scientist. [pause] Assess it [long pause, then her fingers entwine] while your unconscious mind can begin or continue to make changes. [pause, then her fingers curl] Tell me what you're feeling in your hands.

I had been talking for quite a while at this point, with only Anna's nonverbal behavior to guide me. You will always want to pay close attention to how your clients' bodies are responding to what you're saying—muscle twitches or spasms in their face, arms, or torso; finger/hand/arm catalepsy or hovering; changes in breathing, pulse, blinking, eye movement or focus; and so on—because it will help you gauge when something significant, something meaningful, is happening. It helps to know, though, just what the "something meaningful" is *about,* so I most often ask. The more detailed the information I have to work with, the more I can be sure of maintaining our concordance and the more nuanced I can be in my suggestions.

Some of my clients can stay in concordance with themselves while talking with me; others find this impossible or impossibly frustrating. When they're not able to give voice to their experience, I'll usually set up some kind of signaling system with them, where they can communicate with me nonverbally.[4] Anna had no trouble talking, so we were able to benefit from the rich, moment-to-moment detail she provided.

A: [very long pause as her fingers separate, and flex, palms facing each
   other] They're heavy.
D: Uh hum.
A: [continues alternately flexing her fingers and making fists] I'm
   thinking of holding a heavy crystal globe
D: Uh huh.
A: I was holding one time for a picture.

I suspect this memory was associationally triggered by my story of
the lifting-glasses dissertation. So much of being a hypnotherapist is
offering opportunities for serendipitous connections and, when they
happen, putting them to intraventive use.

D: Uh huh. And when was that picture taken?
A: I was young, [her head turns slightly from side to side] I was
   modeling, I was eighteen, nineteen. [pause, then her fingers continue
   to open and close] My hands, it was really for hands, but my face was
   behind the crystal ball. It was heavy and smooth and hard to hold.
   [brings her hands together and entwines her fingers]
D: Uh huh. And can you hold that now?

Anna was describing the picture-taking as a past-tense, long-ago
event, which kept intact the Cartesian split between the rememberer
and whatever is remembered. My question was an invitation for her
to bridge this gap, to get inside, to live, the experience in the present—
to become of one mind with it.

A: They made me take my rings off.

Had she accepted my present-tense invitation, she would have said,
"They *are making* me take my rings off." But she didn't, so I tried
again.

D: [her hands return to her lap] Uh huh. And if you were to look in
   that crystal ball right now, [her fingers entwine] what do you see?

Instead of directly suggesting that she "*look into* the crystal ball,"
I eased her into the possibility of it by more tentatively wondering,

*"if you were to look . . ."* Note, though, that I had dumped the tenta-
tiveness by the end of the question. I didn't ask, ". . . what do you
*suppose you might* see?" but just, ". . . what do you see?" Also, did you
catch the switch in the sensory modality? I thought she might find it
easier to begin by seeing, rather than feeling, the experience.

A: [pause] A lens on the other side, [the tips of her right and left
    index fingers touch each other] of the camera, and my face [pause]
    a flash.

She didn't use a verb in her description, so I wasn't sure how she was
relating to the experience. Was she inside it, living it in the moment,
or still outside it, remembering it in the past? I decided to go for
broke. Taking her description as an in-the-moment account, I seized
on the camera flash as an opportunity for something new to happen.

D: And with that flash, [her fingers separate] de-focus and let the
    image in the crystal ball go blurry for a moment. [pause as her left
    hand cradles the right] And now when you're looking again, look
    at your hands through the crystal ball, and now what do you see?
    [her fingers entwine, lightly rubbing each other, as she lifts her
    hands up near her face]

By suggesting a dis- and then a re-orientation, I was offering Anna
the possibility of noticing something different about her hands. I was
careful, though, to leave it to *her* to discover what the change would
be. When you and your clients are of one mind, the innovation of
your intraventions belongs to both of you. Like any creative brain-
storming, the sparks fly as a result of your *interaction.*

A: [pause] I see my hands and my red nails. [fingers continue to move]
D: Uh huh.
A: And the bones.
D: You can see through the skin?
A: [nods] Yeah, I can see the bones.

Marvelous, eh? I wouldn't have thought of this on my own, and had
*I* attempted to determine what she'd be able to see, the image might

not have fit for her. Far better for you to sketch outlines and designate possible shadings and colors, freeing up your clients to do the fine brush work and make their own creative choices.

D:  And how do the bones look? [each of her hands stretches fingers of opposite hand]
A:  [pause] Knobby.
D:  Uh huh. [pause] Like good strong hand bones? [her fingers, entwined, gently massage and stretch each other]

I was getting too far ahead of her. I might have been better off saying something like, "Tell me more," or "Knobby in what way?" or "How do they look between the knobby parts?"

A:  [pause] They're kinda frail. They need to get stronger.
D:  Uh huh. And look at the muscles on the bones for a minute. What do you see there?
A:  [pause as her fingertips touch up near her face] I don't see any muscles. I just see skin and bone.

I took this to be another statement about the fragility of her hands. She had told me that the bones needed to get stronger, so I figured, "Why not now?"

D:  Ahh. Take one of the fingers now, looking in the crystal ball, and strengthen the bone in one of them. [pause, then her fingertips press against each other and fingers curl] And when you've done that you can tell me.

This intravention was certainly a risk. She might well have said, "The bone is too porous—I can't strengthen it," but if she had, I would simply have looked for another way for the bone to become stronger, suggesting she soak it in a calcium-rich elixir or something. Every suggestion you offer is a kind of experiment. If your clients can take and do something creative with it, then you use whatever change they make in response to it as the jumping-off point for your next suggestion. If they reject it, then you back up and explore other ways of introducing and nurturing change.

I lowered the risks for Anna and me, though, by limiting the scope of my suggestion to one finger. Strengthening one bone would certainly be easier than strengthening all the hand bones at once, and I assumed that if she were successful with this initial small step, she'd have no trouble extending her skill elsewhere.

A: [pause] I think I made it better.
D: Uh huh. And the bone is stronger now? [her fingertips continue touching, then each hand gently stretches fingers of opposite hand]

She said she *thought* she had made it better, so I wanted to confirm that it had "really" happened before proceeding.

A: [nods slightly] Uh huh.
D: And now, what do the muscles look like in *that* finger?

I was implying that her ability to strengthen the bone would allow her, now, to see the muscles. She let me know that I was again moving too fast.

A: [pause while index fingers touch] I have to *put* muscles under the skin.
D: Yeah. You might see the blood vessels first.
A: Uh huh. [fingers stay entwined]
D: And the nerves.
A: Mmm, yeah. [index fingers touch and push against each other]

I was only halfway in sync with her. I got the hint that the muscles were going to take their own sweet time arriving, so I suggested that the blood vessels and the nerves might appear first. So far so good. But I didn't pick up on her saying that she would have to *put* the muscles there. Had I been more attuned to her correction of me, I would have responded differently, speculating about what she would need to *do*, rather than just to *notice*: "You might need to put the blood vessels in place first, and then lay the nerves in." After she had accomplished this, the next step would have been obvious and easy: "Are you ready to attach the muscles, now?"

D: Yeah. So how does that finger now move different from the other
  ones?

My question presumed a difference and allowed her to define what
it was.

A: Now, it's more alive. It's not like a skeleton. [nods]
D: Ahh, [pause] more alive, not like a skeleton.
A: [pause while fingertips touch] It breathes.
D: Ahh, it breathes. [her fingers entwine and return to her lap]

These simple affirmations of her experience furthered our being of
one mind—we were unanimous about what was happening.

When your clients stop marking the difference between you and
them, they are not, as is commonly supposed, submitting to your
will or letting you control them. They are simply finding it unnecessary, for a period of time in a particular context, to differentiate
themselves from you. As you and they develop your rhythmic and
ideational connection—your concordance—they continue to draw
lots of distinctions. How could they perceive or think without them?
But, for the most part, they won't find it necessary to bother attending to the distinction between you and them, between their mind
and body, or between their "self" and other distinguished parts of
their experience (pain, memories, shame, etc.).

When the concordance of these various relationships is intention-
ally or unintentionally interrupted—such as when you need to bring
the session to a close, or in the event that your clients feel threatened,
suspicious, or in any other way out of sync with you or some aspect of
their experience—then the boundaries of ordinary consciousness will
be reasserted, and the trance will end.

D: Can you find another finger? Which finger was that? [she raises her
  right index finger] Can you let its partner in on the [she touches her
  left index finger with her right]—that's right, that one. Can you let
  it breathe as well?

Once change is happening, I look for ways to encourage and extend it.

A: [nods] Yeah, it needs those blood vessels. [pause and then nods
   again]
D: So, put them there, [she nods then lifts her hands, fingers touching,
   up near her face] all the blood vessels it could possibly need, [pause
   as her fingers entwine] and all the muscles it needs, [pause as her
   fingertips touch] and when you're finished with that finger, let me
   know.

Give your clients time to *experience* the present change before inviting
them to take the next step. And wait until you know they're with you
before taking the next step yourself.

A: [long pause and then she nods]
D: Now, do those two fingers feel heavier or lighter than the others?

Erickson would have called this a "therapeutic double bind"[5] or an illusion of alternatives (Erickson & Rossi, 1980). My question offered
Anna the freedom of choice or discovery at the level of the particular
options being offered—whether her fingers felt heavier or felt
lighter—but it *constrained* her ability to choose or discover at the
level of the *set* of options offered. That is, by going in search of an answer to my question, Anna necessarily accepted, unquestioned, the
parameters I had placed on it—her fingers would feel different in *some*
way.

Remember the case I described in the Introduction? When Joannie,
the pregnant woman with excruciating pain in her arms, told me, in
hypnosis, that her arms were full of poison, I commented on how fortunate she was that the problem was poison-related, since this meant
she could just go ahead and let the necessary antidote enter her system. I then explained that I wasn't sure what would happen next:
"I don't know if the antidote will cause the poison to evaporate
through your pores . . . or to drip out the ends of your fingers . . .
or to neutralize it in some other way. Let's let the antidote begin
working and see how the poison changes." Connecting these specific
possibilities was the unstated premise that the antidote would be effective in *some* way. The possibilities I discussed laid out a therapeutic double bind: whichever option proved to be the case, it would be
of benefit to Joannie.

I don't think it makes sense to describe such choices as *illusory.* Anytime you exercise your free choice at one level, you are accepting without question the *fact of the choice,* that is, the connection between (or the set containing) the options. Allow me to illustrate this with a nontherapy example. Let's say you're at your favorite restaurant, and you're trying to decide which entree you want to order. As you go back and forth between the various possibilities, you are determining for yourself that you will eat *some entree.* But what if you're not sure how hungry you are? You'll then try to decide whether to choose one of the smaller entrees or to order an appetizer as the main part of your meal. As you exercise your freedom of choice with regard to the *size* of the portion, you are fixing in place your decision to eat *some portion.*

Let's take this a step or two further. Say you start wondering whether you're hungry enough to eat at all. Perhaps you will just have a glass of wine. By freely choosing between eating and drinking, you are determining that you will *ingest something.* And if you then question whether you want to order anything at all or just sit and talk with your friends, you are then fixing in place that you will be *sitting at the table.* And so on.

Life is full of this inter-level interplay between freedom and determination. So where's the illusion? You can't exercise choice at one level without being subjected to constraints at the next, without accepting (and thus being limited by) the *set of options* from which you are choosing. Every act of freedom is limited by the parameters that determine or define it, and the act itself helps to establish what the parameters are.[6]

A: [her index fingers separate from each other for a few moments and then touch again] Heavier. They're stronger.

Anna was developing an enriched sense of how healthy fingers feel: they breathe, they're heavy, they have blood vessels and strong bones and muscles and nerves. I tied these all together via another double-bind question.

D: Yeah. [long pause] So can you take each of those fingers, and I don't know if they will communicate how to do that to the other fingers [her hands, fingers entwined, return to her lap] on their own hand or whether they'll communicate to the fingers on the opposite hand, but bring life and blood vessels and breath and nerves to all the other fingers. [her hands begin gently massaging each other] And when they're all feeling heavier and more alive, [pause] when they're all feeling that way, let me know.

A: [long pause as her fingertips gently press against each other] Hmmm. [nods as she separates her hands, flexing her fingers]

D: Okay, and that includes your thumbs?

A: Uh huh. [her fingers, pointing up, flex and move]

D: Now, look into the crystal ball again and de-focus, [pause] and refocus in a month from now: [long pause as her fingertips touch and her fingers curl] May 12th, 11th, or 13th. And now what do you see?

If the de- and re-focusing in the ball could give her x-ray vision, why not future vision? By taking her forward a month to see what was happening then, I was implicitly suggesting that the changes would endure.[7]

A: [long pause as her fingers entwine, separate, and then touch] My complete eighteen-year-old hands, nineteen-year-old hands. They're strong.

D: [pause] Hmm.

A: Straight. [fingers entwine and bend back the fingers of the opposite hand]

D: They're complete and strong and straight. [long pause as her fingertips gently push against each other] Now, will you defocus again into the crystal ball, [her hands return to her lap and her fingers entwine] and refocus however long ago, [pause] at a time when your hands were strong and straight and full of life and vigor, [pause] and when you can see that and feel that in your hands, let me know.

If she could reorient in the future, she could also reorient in the past. Both can be useful for establishing resources for change.

A: [very long pause as her fingertips touch, press against each other, and curl]

D: [she nods] Okay, where are you?

This time she responded in kind to my use of the present tense:

A: [reaches up and scratches her right ear with her right index finger]
In my grandmother and aunt's house in the kitchen. [her hands
return to her lap, and she continues slowly entwining and
separating her fingers] My aunt's putting nail polish on my hands.
I'm about four.

D: What color?

A: Red.

D: Hmm. Is she admiring your hands?

A: [nods and smiles] Yeah.

D: And you can feel how full of life they are?

A: Yep. They're cute little hands.

I was asking her merely to confirm her ability to feel a change that
had already occurred. Her hands were full of life—could she tell?
Even if she'd said *no,* I could have backed up and said something like,
"Well, so go ahead and just feel their breathing, and feel the muscles
and nerves and strong bones, and you might even feel how pliable
they are. And now what do you notice?" This would have eventually
gotten us to the same place.

D: Hmm hmm.

A: It's hard to keep them still so she doesn't get the nail polish on the
skin. [right hand rubs behind right ear and then returns to lap and
clasps left fingers]

D: Ahh. 'Cause they're always moving?

A: 'Cause I want to look at it before she's done.

D: Hmm hmm. You're excited?

A: [nods slightly]

D: Is this the first time you've gotten nail polish?

A: No. My grandmother did it once and she got it all over my skin,
and I cried, till my aunt took it off.

D: But this time it's going on right?

A: Hmm hmm. [nods and smiles]

D: Hmmm. And your hands feel wonderful, [she nods] and tingly, and
warm. [her hands separate, palms down; her fingers open and
become still]

A:  And sweaty.

D:  Yeah. [she smiles slightly and nods]

A:  They're on the kitchen table.

D:  Hmm, is it cool?

A:  Smooth. [her right palm lightly rubs her leg]

D:  Uh huh.

A:  It was cool, now it's sticky.

D:  Hmm hmm. And they're *cute* little hands.

I said this (which, you'll recall, was originally *her* description of her hands) with a talking-to-a-four-year-old tone of voice, providing another contextual cue in support of her age regression.

A:  [her fingers wiggle as her hands come together] They still have
    dimples.

I next invited her back to the future, but to an older age than the previous time.

D:  [pause while her left fingers take hold of right index finger] Now,
    de-focus again into the crystal ball, and take those hands forward
    [pause] until you're fifty. [long pause] That's right. And holding the
    crystal ball with those strong hands [pause] at fifty. [long pause,
    then she entwines her fingers and her hands lift up to her chin] And
    what do you see?

A:  [pause while her fingertips push against each other] Lady's hands.

D:  Uh huh. What else? [her fingers remain still]

A:  [pause] Dimples are inside.

I heard this as a sign that, without my asking her explicitly to do so, she had brought into the future the life essence of her childhood hands. Once I had confirmed this impression, I linked the dimples to the images and sensations that she'd earlier associated with her hands feeling strong and healthy.

D:  Uh huh. [her hands alternately massage each other] And the inside
    dimples are keeping them feeling young [pause] and healthy? [she
    smiles slightly] Is that right?

A: Yeah.

D: And you can see those dimples through the crystal ball, but to the normal gaze they'd be invisible, is that right?

A: Right.

D: [her fingers curl] And can you also see then the strong bones and the blood vessels and the nerves?

A: [nods] Yeah. [her fingertips touch and her head comes forward and down until her face touches her hands]

With her hands feeling so good at fifty, I figured we should go still further into the future, bringing the dimples along for the ride.

D: [pause] Yeah. De-focus again, [pause as her head lifts] and now refocus at those seventy-year-old hands, [pause as her fingertips, pointing up, continue to touch] again locating the internal dimples.

A: [long pause] They're really different. [her index fingers touch her nose]

D: Uh huh.

A: [her fingers move away from her face and entwine] The outside's like a shell.

D: Uh huh. In what way? [her hands, fingers entwined, massage each other]

A: Hard and brittle and holding the life and the softness inside.

D: Uh huh. So they're still full of life and softness on the *inside*.

A: Yeah, [nods slightly] like a clam. [her head moves forward until her nose touches her fingers]

D: Uh huh. And they still have that youthful vigor?

A: [her head lifts and she nods] Yeah. They just don't look as good. [her hands, fingers entwined, massage each other]

D: Uh huh. They don't look like the four-year-old hands on the *outside*.

By emphasizing the word *outside,* I highlighted the external/internal distinction that had been in the air since Anna had told me about her fifty-year-old lady's hands having dimples on the *inside.* I hoped that by my saying, "They don't look like four-year-old hands on the *outside,*" she would complete the other half of the distinction on her own, finding herself thinking, "But they still look/feel like them on the *inside.*"

A: They look like my grandmother's hands. [her fingers entwined, she
stretches them by pushing her palms outward]

D: Uh huh.

A: But they work. [her hands, massaging each other, rest in her lap]

D: And they're still strong?

A: [long pause and then she nods] They're strong.

We could now return to the present.

D: [long pause] Yeah. Now look once more, if you would, into the
crystal ball and de-focus [pause as her right leg crosses her left; her
right forearm and hand rest on her right leg, her left hand rests,
palm down, on her right arm] and refocus back to now. [pause as
each hand flexes a little] That's right. And locate those internal
dimples, [pause] that source of life and movement, [pause as her
right hand makes a fist and then relaxes; the fingers of both hands
wiggle a little] and holding tightly to that, tell me what you see.

A: [pause as her hands clasp in her lap] My hands are baby hands
inside.

D: [long pause] Yeah. And what does that bring your hands in order
to be able to see and to feel that?

What a lousy question! She, of course, didn't know what to make of it.

A: [fingers entwine] What?

D: What does that *change* in the feeling of your hands in order to be
able to see and to feel that?

Still a muddy question, but she at least was able to do something
with it.

A: [forty-second pause as her hands massage each other, flex, and
entwine] Um, my hands are pudgier. Softer.

D: Uh huh. [pause] Stronger?

A: Yeah, stronger, straighter, [long pause] smoother.

D: Hmm. And how do they *feel?*

A: [pause as she entwines fingers and brings her hands up near her
face] Hotter.

She said this so softly, I didn't catch the word.

D: [she momentarily rests her chin on her hands] Hotter or harder?
A: Hot.
D: And that heat's bringing them *what?*

When your clients describe a change, inquire, if you can, about the implication it brings. The more detailed information you have, the better you can help vivify their experience.

A: [she alternately flexes her fingers and forms them into fists] Cooking blood vessels. [pause as she entwines her fingers] Makes them more comfortable.
D: [pause] Uh huh. [with her fingers still entwined, her hands return to her lap] Can you take that warmth now and put it in all of the joints in your body?
A: [her fingers remain entwined in her lap; after forty-five seconds, she smiles] They're colder now.

I was applying the same principle as before, using a small change in one place as a jumping-off point for more extensive changes elsewhere. Just as the transformation in one finger can be transported to others, so, too, the transformation in the joints of the hands can be transported to those in the rest of the body.

D: Hmm. [with her fingers entwined, her hands massage each other] And your other joints?
A: They're warmer, except my toes.
D: Hmm. And can you take that, those internal dimples? [pause] And make sure there's an internal dimple [pause] there at every joint.

This was a good next step, but if I could do it over, I wouldn't have proceeded until we'd made sure her toes, too, felt warm.

A: [her hands remain entwined, motionless, and relaxed for three minutes; she then swallows, her lips tighten for a moment, and she stretches a little]

I waited and watched, making sure I didn't interrupt whatever was happening within her concordance with herself. When she swallowed, tightened her lips, and stretched, I assumed she was done, but, before going on, I asked for confirmation.

D: Are you finished?
A: [nods]
D: Good. [pause] And what difference has that made?

I used present-perfect tense ("has made") to help underscore the assumption that something significant had occurred.

A: [long pause as her fingers, entwined, stretch and massage each other] I have my little baby body in me.
D: [long pause] Hmm.
A: And I have more supple muscles.
D: Yes. [long pause as she continues massaging various fingers] What else?

The more details you ask for, the more you encourage your clients to enrich their experience. I want to make sure I don't miss anything, so I'm always asking my clients if they've anything else to tell me. You never know—the tidbit they initially thought not worth mentioning might prove pivotal in turning things around.

A: I can run without thinking about it.
D: Hmm.
A: Just moves, everything just moves. I don't have to pay attention.
D: Yeah. They know how to move on their own?
A: [pause, then nods] . . . .

I next (in a part of the transcript not included here) spent some time talking directly to her fingers, encouraging them to take their newly acquired knowledge and spread it to all other joints in her body. Then, wanting to provide a buffer—relational freedom—between Anna's expectations and any present and future alterations in perception and function, I suggested that she might find the changes surprising. Before bringing the session to a close, I returned to her image of the dimples as a symbol of healthy, comfortable functioning.

D: And you can keep those internal dimples placed at each joint.
A: [long pause, then takes a deep breath and entwines her fingers]
D: And now in your own time you can come back to this room, returning from trance, leaving there what's best left there in trance, and return to the room and the rest of your day feeling rejuvenated and rested.

By drawing a boundary between trance and non-trance, you underscore the distinctiveness of your clients' hypnotic experience, protecting it from the analytic scrutiny of their conscious awareness.

A: [long pause, then her eyelids flutter and open]
D: Hi.
A: Hi.
D: So, how was this one different?

I didn't ask how the experience had *been* for her but how it *differed* from previous sessions. Given that your clients' critical intelligence, like yours and mine, depends on distinguishing *this* from *that,* you might as well put it to work noticing changes and positive developments.

A: This one was a lot brighter. I mean, I saw things very clearly, and, um, I could listen to you and still daydream. [nods] I didn't have to do everything you said, either. Sometimes you were saying something and I was somewhere else.
D: Good.
A: And so it felt more, [pause] it was comfortable to do two things at once.
D: Uh huh. Great.
A: It was like two dimensions at the same time.

At the beginning of our next (and last) session, Anna felt considerably better. The pain in her fingers had "subsided to a tolerable level," and she had "more energy," was sleeping better, and had "a better outlook." And with the pain in her fingers now "minimal," Anna had become less worried about the symptoms getting worse. Asked how we could best use our last meeting, she said she would like to learn more about practicing self-hypnosis. When I suggested that she go ahead and, on her own, develop a hypnotic relationship with herself, she protested, saying she'd never done that before. I disagreed:

> D: Well, actually you have. You see . . . [hypnosis is] just me . . . relating back to you how you're doing this. It is your doing self-hypnosis always, and I provide some violin accompaniment, but it's you that's soloing. So why don't you do that again . . . and I'll provide a little bit of continued commentary about how you can carry this on if you wish on your own without any violins.

By teaching your clients self-hypnosis and giving them the confidence to proceed on their own, you free them up from needing you.

I suggested that Anna didn't need me to provide the accompaniment for her to develop concordance with herself; she could, instead, rely on all the sounds of her outer and inner environment, whatever thoughts she might have, the feelings in her muscles and fingers, her breathing and how it changed, and any other changes going on in her body.

My five sessions with Anna were videotaped as part of a research project I conducted with Sandra Roscoe in 1993.[8] As part of the research protocol, Sandra met with Anna for two followup interviews—the first, eight months after the last session; the second, eight months after that. During the first interview, Anna remembered feeling better toward the end of our hypnosis sessions. But shortly thereafter, she said, she began to get bothered by an old injury to her achilles tendon. After getting some physical therapy for it, she "turned to the same automatic process" that she relied on during our hypnosis sessions. "Okay," she had said to her heel, "we've done the best we can for you now. You're going to get better and I'm not going to interfere with you anymore—no more invasive procedures."

Prior to the second follow-up interview, Anna experienced a flare-up of painful joints.

A:  My first response was, "Oh, just ignore it, it'll go away." And
    sometimes that worked, but when it wasn't working I continued
    to do it, and saying, "Well, any day now. It'll go away, it'll go away,
    it'll go away." I had thought that I would have found something else
    to do after the ignoring part was not working. Either it would work
    or I would do something else. But I was still in a control mode. "I
    can control this if I ignore it. It will go away if I ignore it."

Although "kind of mad that this could happen" when she had been
getting "healthier emotionally and supposedly physically," she nevertheless started practicing self-hypnosis.

A:  Once or twice a week I would go into trance . . . with a global sort
    of question like, "How can I connect to what's happening here?" or
    "What do my fingers have to say?" or "What do my hips have to say
    to me?"

She started to look to see how she could "simplify her life," where she
could "ease up without it being too much."

A:  And if you look, if you really look at it, you can find those places. I
    hadn't been looking at it because I kicked back into "let's just deny
    all this and it'll go way," which works sometimes, but doesn't work
    at other times.

Even though her pain had not gone away completely, Anna described
it as "minor" and "subsiding," and she was again starting to feel
better.

# 6

# Your Clients' Relationship with Their Problem

The patient comes to you and says, "Get rid of my headache for me; get rid of my broken arm for me; get rid of my cancer for me; remove all these distresses from me; I want freedom from my stomachache." . . . They . . . come in with the fundamental attitude that you are going to *abolish* certain things. You should abolish this severe headache, or this aching back, or the pain in that broken leg, when actually, what ought you to do? I tell a patient: "Now, you have rather a bad headache there. I think you ought to make some kind of use of it."

*—Milton Erickson*

It seems that if I am afraid, then I am "stuck" with fear. But in fact I am chained to the fear only so long as I am trying to get away from it.

*—Alan Watts*

Staying loose, allowing yourself the freedom to ramble, opening yourself up to outside influences, keeping a flexible mind willing to entertain all sorts of notions and avenues—this is the attitude that is most appropriate for the start of any project where the aim is to generate something new.

*—Denise Shekerjian*

Take chances, make mistakes, and get messy!

*—Miss Frizzle*

Despite what the DSM—with its cataloging of psychological ailments—implies, no problem exists in isolation, separate from the context of people's experience. Most of your clients, though, make DSM-like assumptions about their problem, thinking of it as if it were a *thing* that, with enough effort and persistence (and the right therapist and perhaps some medication), might be successfully controlled or eradicated. No wonder they arrive in your office feeling exhausted and discouraged. How long have they been failing to dissociate from whatever's been eating at them, failing to put a stop to the problem or to better steel themselves against it?

Your ability to help depends to a significant degree on your recognizing that divisive actions taken to ensure a problem's absence only maintain and underscore its presence. With such a relational understanding, you won't sign on to help your clients keep in check or banish a problem, or even to change it. Rather, you'll act so as to facilitate *a change in their relationship to it.*[1] If your clients' dissociative attempts to negate what they hate have created a *separated connection* with it—a negative relationship that has maintained, or even heightened, its significance—then your job is to facilitate the associative development of a *connected separation:* a relationship with the problem that allows for a comfortable connection and/or a relaxed letting go. Instead of helping to push your clients' problem away, you'll explore ways they can embrace and/or lose track of or interest in it, allowing it to become boring or irrelevant or otherwise unremarkable.

Just in case you're sometimes tempted to dole out Ann Landers' advice to your clients, let me quickly point out that you can't just say to your clients ten minutes (or even ten sessions) into knowing them, "It seems to me that you've been trying to keep these anxiety attacks (or temper fits or depressive episodes or unruly kids or sexual difficulties or nightmares or headaches or whatever) at arm's length. What you need to do, instead, is to become one with them. Just embrace them and then everything will work out just fine." Therapy isn't the equivalent of commanding with Shakespearean authority, "Get thee to a Buddhist monastery!" Rather, it's a matter of helping clients relate to their problem in a different way. You won't accomplish this by *directing* them to think, emote, or act differently, but you *can* offer opportunities that, if they take you up on them, will likely result in a changed relationship to, and a resultant shift in, the problem.

In this chapter, I talk about how you can bring a relational sensibility and sensitivity to your work with client problems. In the first section, I talk primarily about how to *orient* yourself to change; in the second, how to *invite* it. But, as in life, you'll find lots of overlap between thinking and doing.

## *Orienting to Change*

Ever attended a meeting where the time allotted was far in excess of what was required to get the work done? Unless you had a wonderfully efficient facilitator or a vocally dissatisfied participant, I bet everyone adjusted the pace of the discussion to fit the schedule—the pre-established expectation of how long you should spend—rather than to fit the need.

Not wanting either my clients or me to settle into the complacent expectation that our work will require a lengthy (or, worse, an interminable) amount of time, I refuse to practice "How-was-your-week?" therapy. From the first phone call, I'm always orienting to change, to the expectation that something significant is about (or, perhaps, has already begun) to happen. I think of this as "What's-different-from-last-week?" therapy. I'll get to the implementation specifics later; here, I'd like to talk about how to construct a context for brief, relational, therapeutic change.

### Commit to Change *and* Continuity
I know several qualitative researchers—Carolyn Ellis, Larry Cochran, Jerry Gale, and others—who've seen their research interviewees make

a desired life change subsequent to a single in-depth conversation about past and present circumstances. In contrast, I know lots of therapists (including me) who've seen their clients *not* make a desired life change following *multiple* in-depth conversations about future possibilities. So what's the deal? How is it that one research interview can give rise to therapeutic transformation, while a host of therapeutic interviews can lead nowhere?

The difference, to my eye, has something to do with how the participants in each setting orient to problems. Researchers aren't trying to effect change, and the people they interview aren't talking with them about how to achieve it. With no stake in doing anything about problems other than to delve into them—along with other important aspects of interviewees' lives—interviewers and interviewees are at liberty to explore how things are and/or have been, rather than how they might be. Such an ambiance of non-demand reflection provides an excellent opportunity for interviewees to connect to their problematic experiences, which can, in turn, free up new possibilities for thinking, feeling, and/or acting differently.

We therapists, in contrast, get paid to get results, so ideas about and hopes for transformation infuse our conversations with our clients. But with such expectations and expectancy in the air, we can get caught up trying to jump-start the future by jump-*stopping* the present, inadvertently encouraging a separated connection between our clients and what they want to leave behind. This shuts down, rather than frees up, change.

Your therapeutic efforts will be less likely to backfire if you help your clients swap their separated connection for a connected separation, inventing ways to *use,* rather than *abandon,* their present circumstances. I'm not suggesting that you should adopt the no-thought-of-change agenda of a qualitative researcher. After all, your clients aren't paying you to study them. But you can attain a freedom similar to a researcher's if you hold onto a *double* agenda, maintaining a commitment to both change *and* continuity.[2] By respecting the integrity, or at least by making contextual sense, of your clients' current situation (however horrible they and/or you consider it to be), you'll feel less inclined to try to rescue them from their crisis by plucking them from its clutches. Instead, your double agenda will allow you, from a position of relaxed curiosity, to help them creatively transform—or find some freedom in—their relationship to their problem.

## Commit to Something (but not Anything in Particular) Happening

A therapist, Geoff, asked me to consult on a case that he thought, until his most recent session, had been going well; however, he now felt lost and unsure about how to proceed. His client—a middle-aged, unhappily married woman—had talked with him at length about leaving her husband. The more details he had heard, the more Geoff had become convinced that divorce was the only way she'd ever realize her potential. With his support, indeed his encouragement, the woman informed her husband that she was leaving him, and then she found an apartment and contacted a divorce lawyer.

When Geoff and his client met for their first appointment after her move into her own place, she told him that she'd decided to give her marriage another chance. She wanted to continue in therapy, either alone, or, if Geoff would agree to it, with her husband; however, she understood, she said, that coming in as a couple might be difficult, given all she'd said during their previous sessions. Caught off-guard and disturbed by her change of mind, Geoff told her he needed some time to think about the best way to proceed. The next day, feeling stuck, he stopped by my office to talk.

After he filled me in on the details, I asked Geoff why he was surprised and what he wanted to do. He sat silently for a long time before replying that his client had seemed so strong and courageous that he never anticipated that she might rethink her decision to end the marriage. He was committed to helping her change, he said, but he was no longer sure she wanted to. He thus wondered whether he should decline to see her at all.

I told Geoff that he sounded committed to his client's changing in a particular trajectory and within a particular time frame. With such an orientation, he would of course interpret his client's seeming U-turn as a failure for both of them. But what if he understood her decision as a move forward, as a further manifestation, rather than a lapse, of her strength? Imagine the courage she must have needed to listen to herself, rather than him, and then to come in and forthrightly tell him of her decision, knowing that he would likely disapprove. Having demonstrated such strength with him, could she not, perhaps, also bring it into her relationship with her husband? If she were to continue to tune into herself, what else would she discover? And if the marriage turned out not to be a good choice for her, could not the strength required to go back also be directed toward leaving again? With these and other questions in mind, Geoff was able to free himself from defining success in terms of only one course of action.

I suspect that Geoff wouldn't have been caught so flat-footed had he had some hypnosis experience. When you're inviting clients into trance or offering them possibilities for experiencing hypnotic phenomena, you commit to *something* happening, but you remain flexible about exactly what that something will be and how and when it will take place. For example, if you asked me to do hypnosis with you, I'd never respond by saying, "When I snap my fingers, your eyelids will close and you won't be able to move your legs or arms." Where would you and I then be if, when I snapped, you kept your eyes wide open, crossed your legs, and scratched your face? By not following my specific demands, you'd be defining yourself in contradistinction to me, maintaining the boundary between us and precluding our being of one mind. Your integrity would be in good shape, but hypnosis with me would be out of the question. I'd be much better off saying something like this, instead:

As I continue to talk, your eyelids may start taking a little rest at the bottom of each blink, extending the time before they open again. Or maybe they'll stop blinking altogether for a while and then all of a sudden spontaneously close. Or they might find their *own* way to feel more comfortable, just as your arms and legs can settle in. Don't be surprised if, at some point, you realize that they feel too relaxed or too heavy to move, so much so that they'd stay put even if you were telling them the opposite.

Ever made a decision to get up and do something but you felt just too deliciously comfortable to get up? Of course, your arms might feel so comfortable, so comfortably independent, that as you sink further and further down into your chair, one or both of them will start to float up.

I once worked with a man whose arms felt glued to the arms of the chair while his feet started feeling lighter and lighter and actually lifted effortlessly off the floor. Who knows whether your eyelids will stay up and your hands will lift up in solidarity with them, your eyelids will sink down and your arms or feet will balance them out by feeling lighter and lighter, or all of you will just sink down, down, down.

This version isn't just longer than the snappy one; it would offer you specific options from which to choose, including the possibility of your body finding its own unique way to proceed. By not nailing down the specifics of your experience, I'd be preserving your freedom to discover that *something,* yet to be defined, could (or perhaps had already started to) happen. Later in the chapter, I'll explain how this way of structuring suggestions builds such expectations. At this point, I just want to highlight the importance of your offering your clients the same freedom of discovery. If, as a therapist, you commit yourself to only one outcome, or to only one kind of outcome, you threaten your relationships with your clients (and their relationships with themselves) when things don't turn out as planned or hoped.

## Approach Problems as Waves
## Rather than Whirlpools

A man who had traveled the Amazon river three times told me about a whirlpool he once saw that had kept a large boat captive for several years. Mist from a high waterfall hung in the air, so a person watching from the shore could see the boat only during the closest arc of its circular path, as it emerged and then disappeared from view. The man had found the eerie sight an unsettling reminder of the river's consuming power, and he wisely kept his distance.

Since the advent of the solution-focused therapy revolution, I've met many therapists who treat client problems as if they were Amazonian whirlpools, capable of trapping hapless helpers in their dizzying suction. Anxiously wanting to adhere to what they believe are the tenets of the solution-focused model, such therapists are loathe to acknowledge their clients' pain or to listen, in any detail, to descriptions of their predicaments. They seem to believe that their job is to pull their clients to safety and that to do so, they must keep themselves distant from the vortex of their problem, allowing discussion only of exceptions and post-miracle futures. Unfortunately, in their scramble to "keep things positive," they fail to recognize that, given the relational nature of mind and language, refusing to talk about something is an ideal way of heightening its significance.

When I encounter solution-drenched therapists, I sometimes tell them a story about one of my clients, a story that provides a different water metaphor to use in organizing their work.

When multiple shots of bourbon prior to and during airplane trips failed to take care of Sandy's panic attacks, he decided to try hypnosis. As usual, I devoted our first session to asking loads of questions about his pre- and in-flight experiences, but also about the other-than-airplane-riding parts of his life. I found out that he was an avid, accomplished surfer who enjoyed the risks and the highs of carving big waves. From the very first time he'd fallen off his board, he said, he'd instinctively known not to fight the undertow. Instead, he would always swim *with* the post-crash riptide until its pull dissipated and he could head to the surface with a minimum of effort. We were able to incorporate his body's grasp of wave dynamics in our hypnotic work, providing him with the ability to board airplanes with the anticipation of a surfer, ready to ride the leading edge of any waves of panic that arose, and ready, if he fell into the crashing swell, to swim down with it, rather than trying to fight it, thrashing his way to the surface. With such preparation, Sandy encountered no further disturbing in-flight swells, and his thrills were restricted to his adventures at the seashore.

I prefer to approach therapy with the sensibility of a surfer, rather than an Amazon explorer. I don't fear being centripetally sucked into my clients' problems; instead, I look forward to diving into them and swimming, like Sandy, downward with the current. Recognizing that by doing this, I'm actually facilitating my return to the surface for my next lungful of air, I'm able to take my time and learn what I need to know about the unique nuances of the situation.

## Trust the Revolutionary Nature of Emotions
Sandy's swimming technique is metaphorically relevant not only for therapists, but also for clients. Rather than viewing my clients' emotional responses as *states of being*—"she is depressed"; "he is angry"; "they are both anxious"—I consider them to be thoughtful, embodied expressions of the clients' relationship with themselves and/or to someone or something else. As such relationships change, so do the associated emotions.

Most of us have been taught to control our emotions—not to give into sadness, to keep our tempers in check, to hold down our fear. Such strategies can work pretty well in the short term for transient emotional responses, but any enduring effort to manhandle our body responses will create a separated connection between the *i*—the Napoleonic part of the self trying to call the shots—and the rogue emotion.

A therapist came to me, asking for a consult on a woman she'd seen three or four times. The client had, several weeks earlier, lost her adult son in a tragic accident and, since then, hadn't been able to stop crying. Her remaining children had been sympathetic at first, but they were now telling her it was time to get on with her life. More importantly, the nonstop crying had swelled her eyes and surrounding tissues to such a degree that her doctor was warning her, with considerable urgency, that her sight was in jeopardy. As a result, the woman had yet another reason to grieve, another reason to cry uncontrollably.

The therapist, overwhelmed by the depth of the woman's pain and concerned about her going blind, desperately wanted to help her. She knew that counseling her to stop or even control the crying would make matters worse, but she saw no alternative.

I suggested talking to the woman about the importance of mourning fully and deeply. Her crying was an understandable response to such a tragic loss, a fitting way of expressing the scale of her despair. Yes, it was dangerous to cry, but how could she not? Rather than following her doctor's and her children's advice, why not listen to her body? She felt the need to wail, so she should. But perhaps she could reach more deeply and cry more thoroughly than she had so far, allowing her tears, whatever the danger to her sight, to express more purely the fierce agony she felt. And the best way for this to happen would be to protect time, perhaps an hour a day, to *concentrate* her grief in the most complete way possible—her doctor and the others be damned. During this hour, she could let the tears flow freely, could *encourage* them to flow plentifully, knowing that this was a necessary, if dangerous, part of her honoring the memory of her son.

Soon after this idea was conveyed to the client, her crying abated considerably (save for the protected hour). The swelling in and around her eyes went down and her sight was saved. By protecting time to cry, she was able to fully enter her grief, allowing the relationship (between her and her emotion) to change.

## Trust Clients' Bodies

As I mentioned in Chapter 5, some therapeutic approaches, such as twelve-step and anger-management programs, are built on the assumption that clients can only protect themselves and others by treating themselves with suspicion. The result is painfully ironic: Any feeling of personal safety (e.g., "I won't take a drink," "I won't lose my temper") is predicated on never feeling safe ("I can't trust that I won't lose control"). Imagine your exhaustion if you could never relax without remaining on guard. I thus prefer to orient toward my clients' trusting themselves, toward trusting (or at least respecting) what their bodies are capable of doing.

When my kids decided they no longer wanted to wear diapers during the day, they stopped peeing at night. Eric was confident about his ability not to wet the bed—he insisted from the start on wearing underwear under his pajamas. Jenna was initially more cautious, requesting for a couple of weeks that we continue putting on a diaper at bedtime. But both of them, once they'd made the daytime switch, were virtually always dry at night. How did their bladders figure out how to make such an instantaneous transition? I don't know the developmental explanation, but I do know that if a two-and-a-half-year-old's body can adapt while he or she is sleeping, then my clients' bodies can make analogous alterations in how *they* work, with an analogous lack of conscious involvement and without the necessity of relentless scrutiny and control.

One of my practicum teams once worked with a woman who was worried that her barely contained anger would soon explode into violence. Recently divorced, she had to work hard to keep her fury in check when her ex-husband picked up their kids for his visitation. More often than not, when our client looked out the window of her house and saw his "cute little girlfriend" in the car, she'd be gripped by the urge to "crush her." She was afraid that if she were to come face to face with her, she wouldn't be able to keep herself from "losing it," so she requested that we help her control her anger or somehow lower it to a safe level.

Counter to her expectations, we talked to her about the productive potential of what she was feeling. She had told us that her ex-husband's leaving her had given her the resolve never to let him get her down. With this in mind, we speculated about the helpfulness of the anger in facilitating such a goal, about how it could help her get to a new place. Knowing that she drove a three-quarter-ton truck, we offered an image that captured the essence of the idea.

> When the two love-birds have been showing up in your driveway, you've been afraid you're going to go out and hurt the girlfriend, right? So your blood pressure skyrockets while you hold yourself back, keeping yourself from doing something that would land you in prison and guarantee that your ex- would get custody of the kids. You've been successful in not losing it, but your method has taken its toll. You don't get any of the short-term benefits that anger offers. It's like flooring the gas pedal of your truck while keeping your left foot firmly planted on the brake. God forbid your left leg should get tired—you'd screech forward and run down whoever was unlucky enough to be in front of you. So that brake foot has been essential in keeping you safe.
>
> But what if you had another way of ensuring your safety? Another way of channeling the anger? What if you kept your right foot pressed to the floor, same as before, but instead of pressing hard with your other foot, you used both hands to spin the steering wheel? You'd send gravel flying, and your ex-husband and his girlfriend would be eating your dust as you showed them your backside and peeled off into your future. Could you do this without your anger? Maybe, but it would take longer.

A big smile appeared on her face when she heard this, and during subsequent appointments, she talked for the first time about getting on with her life. No longer afraid of her anger, she was able to welcome it as a vehicle of change rather than of destruction—a way of screeching away from her ex-husband in a satisfying, let-'em-eat-dust sort of way.[3]

## Facilitate Change in Relationships

I knew a woman whose marriage disintegrated while we were both completing our master's degrees in counseling psychology. Her experience with her divorce proved unsettling for her personally, of course, but it also had a significant effect on her professionally. She had entered the master's program believing she could learn to change people, but her personal ordeal had shaken her hope and sullied her ideals. Despite her diligence in attempting to bring out the best in her husband, he had remained the same stubborn, sexist S.O.B. as when she first met him. This had led her to conclude that "no one ever really changes" and, therefore, that therapy is a crock. Last I heard, she'd gone back to school to pursue a new career.

If I'd had the understanding and experience at the time to challenge my classmate's assumptions, I'd have pointed out that therapy isn't about *changing people,* it's about *facilitating change in relationships*—the relationships clients have with themselves, each other, and their problems. Clients may, as a result of such changes, feel like they have become a new or different person, but that's the stuff of personal reflection and evaluation, not therapeutic intent. I simply look for ways that separated connections can be transformed into connected separations, for ways that constricted relationships can be freed up.

## Be an Advocate for Learning
## Rather than Winning

Consider the role of cheerleaders at sporting events. They clamor for their team when someone makes a great play, and they root for it when someone falters. At all times, their ambient bubbly enthusiasm proclaims the idea, "Come on! You can do it! You can win!"

No wonder, then, that some therapists have adopted such an approach as part of their arsenal of techniques. If cheerleading helps elite athletes, why not clients?

But I'm not a fan of the idea. I've seen too many therapists limit their freedom by getting firmly and vocally behind only signs of "positive change." If you cheer excitedly when your clients do well, what's left to do when they don't? Mask your disappointment and murmur "chin-up" encouragements? Instead of acting amazed and excited when clients tell me about a positive development in their situation,

I offer my sincere *interest*—the same interest I extend when they tell me about a rough patch, a "bad" choice, or an intensification of the problem. Regardless of the direction of their change, I stay curious about how it will contribute to the range and depth of their experience.

This means that, rather than implicitly setting therapy up as a context for winning, I explicitly establish it as a laboratory for trial-and-error learning. My clients and I conduct mini-experiments, allowing them to get as much or more from experiences that bomb as from those that go swimmingly. As a result, failures are always relative and necessary. And the lousy choices and dangerous mistakes they make outside the focus of our therapeutic work are helpful in the same way—essential for creative transformations. In all cases, recognizing that learning is impossible if they're busy recoiling from themselves (see Chapter 5), I invite their curiosity about their situation. To introduce the idea of trial-and-error change, I sometimes tell a story about the time Shelley helped me allow Eric to crash his bicycle.

Several times a week, Shelley and I go for a forty-minute run on the streets of our neighborhood. Jenna still accompanies us in a jogging stroller, but for the last couple of years, Eric has been riding alongside us on his bicycle. He manages well now, but when we first started letting him pedal with us, he drove us crazy. He's always liked riding fast, and he has a penchant for searching out and heading for any bump, pothole, or chunk of debris he can find. As I ran, I was constantly on edge, telling Eric to slow down, watch where he was going, be careful, listen for cars, and on and on. While Shelley would push the jogging stroller, I'd "ride herd" on Eric, making sure to run along beside him so that when he lost control, I could keep him from splatting all over the road. He wore a helmet, of course, but I was still worried about hard falls, about broken arms or bloody scrapes. I wasn't having any fun, and neither was anyone else.

One day, as I was lacing up my shoes, bracing myself for the day's obstacle-course adventure, Shelley looked at my clenched jaw and started laughing at me. "You're funny—you never tell your clients to stop doing what they're doing, even if it's dangerous. You find out how it fits for them and then let them figure out the best decision for themselves. How come you're not doing the same for Eric? Let him fall! That's the only way he's going to learn to control the bike himself."

As (almost) always, she was right. My protecting had precluded his learning. With a shudder and a deep breath, I accepted that, by facilitating a few minor spills now, I'd be able to help prevent major ones later on. I continued protecting him from cars and other major threats to his life, but I allowed him the freedom to discover, in classic trial-and-error fashion, how to protect *himself*. I held back and let him crash. And crash again. And again. Finally he started paying attention to what he was doing—something I'd been trying, but miserably failing, to promote.

Let me tell you a few other stories that similarly demonstrate the benefits of adopting a pro-learning, as opposed to a pro-positive-change, position.

Loni brought her eighteen-year-old son, Stefan, to our university clinic, hoping the therapist I was supervising could "make him more responsible." Planning to move across the country in a few months, Loni wanted Stefan to continue living with his grandmother, helping her remain independent in her own house. Stefan liked the plan, but Loni had begun to doubt whether he was up to the task. He drove like a maniac, he was bar hopping at night, spoiling for fights, and he had recently been fired from a construction site after grabbing his boss and threatening to throw him down a half-finished flight of stairs.

Working together with one of the therapists on my team, I talked to Stefan about possibilities for his future. He wanted, he said, to get his temper under control, and he'd like to be able to keep a job. But mostly he wanted his mom to get off his back. Loni was hoping we would admonish him to grow up, as if hearing it from us would make more of an impression than it had coming from her. I decided to try making a different kind of impression.

DOUGLAS: Have you ever heard, Stefan, of the martial artists who claim to be able to penetrate their hand in under their opponent's sternum? They say they can drill in under the rib cage with the tips of their fingers, reach up, grab the heart, rip it out, and hold it up for the guy to see before he drops dead.
STEFAN: [shakes his head *no*.]
D: Your mother wants you to change. She wants us to make you more responsible. But that's impossible. You might never change. Nobody can stop you from losing your temper, threatening your

bosses, looking for fights at night, or driving like crazy. If you change, it will be because *you* decide you don't want to keep living this way, but it won't be because of us or your mom.

I don't know what it will take for you to decide you're going to make different choices. Could be that you'll have to actually send a boss down a set of stairs. Not just threaten to push him, but actually *shove* him down. Maybe when you hear the crack of his skull on the fresh concrete edge of a step, maybe the sound will help you decide you want to do something different with your anger. Or maybe it won't happen until after you see him lying in a heap at the bottom, his head leaking blood, his arm bent backwards at an impossible angle, that you'll change.

Or maybe you'll have to get into a knife fight outside a bar and it will be the feel of the knife slicing into the other guy's belly that will start you down a different path. The feel of the slight resistance just before the blade pierces the skin, and then the fast plunge to the hilt. Or maybe it will be the gushing of the blood when you pull the knife out, gushing all over your hand and arm and legs and feet. Maybe the sticky warmth of the blood will do the trick.

Or it might be that you have to go to prison for the attempted murder of the guy at the bar, and in your twentieth year there, angry and middle-aged, you'll finally decide that when you get out you'll treat yourself and treat others differently. Or maybe prison itself won't be enough. Maybe you'll have to get into a bunch of fights over the years and only when you finally kill a guy with your bare hands, only when he slumps down in front of you, his eyes glazed, will something inside of you shift and you'll say to yourself, "This is bullshit, I don't need this shit anymore." Or maybe it will be when he kills you. As you slide to the floor and the room starts spinning and the pain is sizzling through you, burning so bad you can't see or think, as your life drains out of you, maybe then you'll have this feeling, this warm understanding that will spread through you, and you'll get this sense that if you'd lived, you'd have made some kind of important change.

Or maybe it won't be a fight that does it. Maybe you'll be speeding tomorrow and too late you'll see a little two-year-old girl with long blonde hair step out in front of you. It may take the slow-motion nightmare of your bumper throwing her up in the air, of her smashing into your windshield, the screeching, opening your door, lifting her into your arms, blood streaming down your arms, looking over there and seeing her mother, in slow motion, running toward you, screaming, "No! No! No!" and the dead weight of the girl in your arms, feeling heavier than anything you've ever felt, maybe it will be the little dead bleeding blonde girl in your arms that makes the difference for you. I don't know what it will be or when it will be, but I know it won't be because of what your mother says to you or what anybody else says. It won't happen according to your mother's schedule but according to yours, according to your making some kind of shift that's yours, no one else's, and that will happen in *your* time and in *your* way.

The other therapist and I stood up at this point and shook Stefan's hand, ending the session. Loni looked less than pleased, but she scheduled another appointment.

I didn't offer my speculations in an effort to be "paradoxical." I certainly didn't want Stefan to have to kill or be seriously injured before he changed course, but I figured that something more dramatic than his mother's lectures would have to happen if he was to reassess where he was headed. I hoped my vivid-as-possible speculations might provide the necessary trial-and-error drama for his making different choices, but I also figured he might need more than a virtual-reality learning experience.

Two weeks later, when they returned, Stefan had two pieces of news. First, he had started driving slowly in their neighborhood. He wasn't sure why, he just had found himself slowing down. Second, he had been at a party across the street from his house on the weekend, and the weirdest thing had happened.

S: I have this reputation in our neighborhood, 'cause I've caused some trouble and stuff, so the parents don't like me. They're scared of me. This lady came up to me at the party, I knew her, but it wasn't her party, and she got in my face and told me to get out. I was pissed. Now normally I would have started yelling at her to mind her own fucking business and maybe I would've grabbed her or given her a little shove or something. Let her know not to mess with me. But for some reason, I didn't do that. I stayed real cool. I don't know how. This feeling just came over me. I didn't get mad. I was real polite. I told her that it wasn't her house so she had no right telling me to leave. If Greta [the mother of the kid whose party it was] didn't want me there, she could tell me, but not you. It was so weird. *She* was the one who lost it. I stayed calm, never raised my voice, and she was the one who started yelling and screaming, and when I didn't react, she stomped out of the house.

Stefan and his mother came back another few times, more for follow-up than therapy, and his changes seemed to stick—enough, at least, for Loni to follow through with her plans to leave. We commented on Stefan's learning, but to preserve our flexibility of response in case he got into further trouble, we didn't cheer his successes. We found them *intriguing*, not *wonderful*.

Another mother, Judith, contacted me late one May, frantic about a son the same age as Stefan, but with a significantly different concern. A bright and universally liked twelfth-grade student, Ben had been accepted by all the universities to which he'd applied, but with eleven days left in his final term, he was on the verge of flunking out. His high school had a strict policy about unexcused absences: If you racked up more than a set number, you automatically failed. Earlier in the day of the evening Judith called me, Ben had reached the magic threshold. If he skipped one more class, he'd lose the year and lose his spot at the university he'd chosen. Terrified that this would launch him on a lifetime path of failure, Judith asked me for an emergency appointment. I agreed to see her and Ben for a two-hour session the next day.

According to Judith, Ben's teachers and his guidance counselor were aware of his precarious situation, and they were all rooting for him to succeed. He'd done so well all year that he wasn't required to take any of the finals, so, as long as he attended all his classes, he'd be fine. Like his mother, his guidance counselor had been lecturing him about the importance of graduating, and his teachers had urged him to come to class, even if he didn't participate. One of them had even given him permission to fall asleep! For the previous several weeks, Judith had been watching with growing frustration and apprehension as Ben's cutting classes had inched him closer and closer to the edge of total failure. Feeling helpless, she was hoping desperately

that I'd be able to get through to him, that my advice would somehow mean more to him than hers, his teachers', his college-bound
friends', and his guidance counselor's.

I wasn't opposed to voicing an opinion, but I wasn't about to join
everyone else in urging him to back away from the ledge he'd built.
Instead, I celebrated his reaching adulthood and the freedom of choice
that goes along with such a transition. I speculated that the question
of whether or not he was going to blow the year had become a lot more
interesting that the stuff he was having to put up in the classes themselves. Now, for the next eleven days, he could wake up with the
choice teetering in front of him. Not often are we so aware of the
degree to which a small, seemingly insignificant, gesture—say, going
or not going to a single class—could determine the rest of our life.

How could he possibly fall asleep at school with such an awareness
alive in him, with such freedom being exercised moment-by-moment?
Anybody urging or demanding or deciding that he should choose only
one of the alternatives would be taking away the choice itself, and with
no choice, his freedom would disappear. With no freedom, he would
lose the electric feeling in his body, and with no electricity, he might as
well go to sleep, resigned to a life of boredom. He had always been such
an excellent student. But didn't he have the right, like anyone else, to
experience and learn from a significant failure?

Failing is a way of learning, but also a way of saving face. What if
he were to not skip any more classes and graduate, only to realize in
the summer that he really wasn't ready to go off to college? Could he,
at that time, go to his mother and tell her he wanted to stay home?
Would she even agree? By failing now, and in such an iconoclastic
way, he'd never have to talk to her about being nervous about leaving. Far better, perhaps, to be a tough rebel than a scared not-yet
freshman. And what if he left, only to realize once he had started the
term that he was over his head? He might find it pretty humiliating
coming home at the end of September. Sealing his fate now would
protect him from not measuring up next fall. Shouldn't he have the
freedom to decide to play it safe by appearing to play it dangerous?
Who wouldn't rather be too bored to bother going to high school
than too scared to try going to college?

He must have been finding it hard, though, to benefit from such a
significant learning opportunity when everyone was telling him what

to do. How could he hear himself think, how could he allow himself to figure out his next step, how could he clearly sort out his options when he was devoting so much of his life to defending his actions?

With Ben's situation laid out as an opportunity for learning, regardless of the choice he made, the high-stakes standoff between him and his mother disappeared. Judith obviously wanted him to go to college, but by the end of the session, she was telling him that she wanted him to make up his own mind. A couple of weeks later, she called to let me know that Ben had stopped skipping classes, had graduated, and was making plans to move in mid-August.

## Know What's Normal

"Should I be worried about this?" Don't we all ask this question—if not explicitly, then implicitly—all the time? And for good reason.

"Is this mole normal, or should I get it checked out?"

"Are the changes in the weather a result of normal variation or of global warming?"

"Are these behaviors of my kids appropriate, given their ages?"

If action is called for but not taken, the result can be disastrous. But if action is taken when it's *not* called for, the result can be equally harmful. With this in mind, I make an effort, whenever possible and appropriate, to normalize the experience of my clients. If you're going to do the same, you'll need to have a general handle on developmental processes and how bodies-and-minds work.

Let me clarify what I mean. I'm not suggesting that you judge your clients according to some normative standard or that you encourage them to adopt more "normal" behaviors and parenting techniques and communication styles. Absolutely not. But I do think it's helpful for you to know, for instance, that as men age, their penis requires more post-orgasm recovery time before being able to become erect again. Or to know that people's inability to remember early childhood experiences has a lot to do with the fact that the brain is still developing during this period. Or to know that having an important person unexpectedly snatched away—by death, by betrayal, by divorce—will heighten the significance of the relationship, making it more likely that the missing person will, at least for a time, figure prominently in dreams and/or daytime reveries. Or to know that because of the nerves connecting the nipples and genitals, a woman, as she's breastfeeding her baby, might well experience some degree of "sexual" arousal (Oxenhandler, 1996).

When you understand how body-and-mind stuff like this works, you'll be less geared up to intervene with clients who are worrying about "normal" body-and-mind responses. Thinking *intra*ventively, you won't set out to "fix" them; instead, you'll look for ways to reassure them that minimal or no action is required.

A mother called me, "worried sick" that her four-year-old boy, Eddie, would grow up to be a rapist. Her concern was sparked by Eddie's "inordinate interest" in her body, as well as some other inappropriate (according to her) sexual-related behaviors. Asked to describe what she'd been noticing, she told me that a few days prior to her call to me, she'd taken a shower, wrapped herself in a towel, and gone looking in her bedroom for some clothes. Eddie was sitting on her bed, and when she asked him to give her some privacy, he offered to hide under the comforter. That way, he explained, he wouldn't see anything, but they'd still be able to talk. She told him that this "wouldn't do," that he needed to give her some peace, whereupon he crawled under the bed. She got him to come out, but when she reiterated her request for him to exit the door, he asked if he could keep it open a crack. Knowing that he'd peek in, she said no.

"Why on earth," she asked me, "would a four-year-old boy be so intent on looking at his mother?" I inquired if they'd recently instituted a new privacy rule in their house. "Oh, yes," she replied, "but in fact in this case it wasn't really modesty or anything—I just wanted some time to myself. But when he refused to go, I got to thinking. He asked his eleven-year-old sister awhile ago if she wanted to see him naked, and he and his three-year-old cousin recently took their clothes off together. I don't think they were touching, though, just looking. And when my daughter and I were going out one night, my son asked my husband, 'Hey Dad, when the girls are gone, do you want to get *naked?*'"

I pointed out that her telling him to leave the bedroom, coupled with the recently instituted give-people-their-privacy rule, had no doubt sparked his interest in the first place: "What cool thing," he'd be asking himself, "is going to happen in here that I'm not supposed to see?" I also noted that rapists are out of relationship with the humanity of the person they are violating. Her son, in contrast, sounded curious about bodies and people—he wanted to talk to her while she got dressed, he wanted to share his newfound body awareness with his sister and cousin, and he wanted to share his "guyness" with his dad. I suggested she talk with her husband about my comments and get back with me if they thought they needed to schedule an appointment. When I touched base with her six weeks later, she told me that everything was fine and she was no longer nervous.

## Think Categorically

Let me begin by juxtaposing three stories.

Carrying a big box of supplies for a booth we were to staff at a family therapy conference, my colleague Chris Burnett and I finally arrived at the exhibit hall, only to find that it had been closed for the evening. The box was too heavy to lug all the way back to my hotel room, and the door to the hall wasn't yet locked, so we opened it, entered, and started looking for our assigned space in the semi-darkness. A security guard, catching sight of us, yelled, "Hey fellas!" but before he could tell us to get out, I called back, "Hi—just bringing in our last load; it will only take a second." He waved us on.

A mother and father brought their five-year-old son, Darryl, in for therapy, worried that he might be seriously mentally ill. In the weeks preceding their coming to see me, Darryl had been regularly snapping the necks of some ducklings nesting on the edge of a canal behind the family's home. The parents had lectured him on the sanctity of life, had punished him, had banished him from the yard, had rewarded gentle behaviors, and so on, but the little birds kept turning up dead, and Darryl "showed no remorse for his actions." Indeed, he seemed to positively delight in the killing.

I suggested to the parents that when they got home from our meeting, they take Darryl out to the canal and help him identify and personally name each of the remaining ducklings. Once they'd agreed on names, they were to begin making up stories, composing a unique tale for each bird. The following week, the parents told me that the killing had stopped completely and that they'd begun to entertain the possibility that their son would not grow up to be an ax murderer.

Ever since his friend's house had been burglarized several months earlier, Robert, eleven, had been terrified of encountering a prowler somewhere in his parents' new two-story house. If the family was upstairs watching television, Robert refused to go downstairs to the kitchen to fetch his mother or father a drink, and if everyone was in the kitchen, he would not, by himself, head upstairs to his bedroom or the family room. He was both frustrated and humiliated by his inability to negotiate the stairway on his own.

Near the end of the first session, I suggested that the therapists seeing the family—Manny and Sandra[4]—help Robert form a concrete picture of the menacing, shadowy presence that was causing him such misery. When asked for a general description of what the person looked like, Robert said he didn't know, that it was "just someone normal." However, he was able (with his eyes closed) to answer a series of specific questions:

SANDRA: Is this burglar a he or a she?
ROBERT: A he.
MANNY: Is he tall or short?
R: Short.
S: Does this short guy have dark hair or light hair?
R: Dark.
M: Does this short dark-haired guy have brown or blue eyes?
R: Brown.
S: Does this short, dark-haired, brown-eyed guy have light or dark clothes?
R: Black, dark clothes.
M: Is he carrying anything or are his hands empty?
R: Empty.

With this now-clear picture constructed, the therapists asked Robert the name of the burglar. He didn't know, so they asked him to keep his eyes closed as they explored various possibilities. "It might be a short name, . . . or it could be a long one. It might be the name his friends call him, . . . or perhaps the one his mother uses. It might be a serious name, . . . or maybe a funny-sounding name. . . ."

"Richard," Robert said suddenly, "His name is Richard."

We ended the session by suggesting that the family go home and sit on the stairs together while Robert drew a picture of Richard.

By the next session, a few weeks later, Robert had, for the most part, "just gotten used to the stairs." We decided it was time for Richard to have a nickname. But what should it be? Rick? Ricky? or Richie? We asked Robert to decide on his own and to draw some more pictures, including one he could carry around in his wallet or shirt pocket. And we asked the parents to find ways to invite Rick or Ricky or Richie into the family—to bring him into conversations, to let him play games and eat meals with them, and so on.

In the third and final session, held six weeks after the first, the family described all the ways they'd made "little Richard" (the nickname they'd settled on) a part of the family. He accompanied Robert on his bicycle ride to and from school, he served as a look-out man on the stairwell, where he would let everyone know that the coast was clear, and he'd acquired a lighter-colored wardrobe. Robert's fear had dissipated almost completely, and his parents noticed how he'd begun to grow up in different areas of his life. We suggested that Robert get Little Richard to help him develop his lay-up and hook shot, and we joked that when it came time to be asking girls out, Robert could ask Little Richard to double-date with him. Robert's comfort at home was still fine six months and a year later; I'm not sure what happened to Richard, but I presume that with his new nickname and duds, great meals, and a family to hang out with, he, too, continued changing in positive ways. And I'm sure that at some point, probably before Robert, he left home.

Okay, so what's with the three stories? All of them illustrate the use and effect of context-creating comments, questions, or suggestions. As I explained in Chapter 1, contexts are established by way of connections, which, in language, involves either metaphor or categorization. I'll get to metaphor in a minute; here, I want to focus on how categories work.

A category is a connection—it links discrete items in terms of one or more shared attributes. You and I are both *readers;* wine, tea, and sparkling water are all *beverages;* cell phones, laptop computers, and pagers are all *portable technological innovations.* Such categories classify—or contexualize—their members, giving them meaning.

When a category is named—"reader," "beverage," "portable technological innovation," whatever—it is available for conscious scrutiny, just like any other isolated item of perception, language, or thought. When a category *isn't* named, it still contextualizes the items it connects, and thus determines their meaning, but it does so invisibly, silently, at the periphery of consciousness.

In each of the situations I described above, the creation of unnamed categories shaped the understanding, experience, and choices of the people involved, without their awareness that this was happening. Milton Erickson termed such offerings "indirect suggestions," but I prefer "context suggestions," as it better captures, I think, the category-creating nature of the process.

When I told the exhibit-hall security guard that Chris and I were bringing in our last load, I made us out to be more legitimate than we actually were. The word *last* categorized our actions as being the end of a series. Given that this was our *last* load, we were obviously *returning* to the hall, which meant that we must have been previously authorized to be there. No need, then, for the guard to worry about us.[5]

Is it possible to perpetrate violence without having first cast the to-be-violated being as Other? I don't think so. Armies get their soldiers in a killing mood by degrading the enemy, characterizing them as less-than-human, as animals or monsters. In contrast, peace negotiators get leaders in a treaty-making mood by elevating the enemy, characterizing them as equally-human, as parents and children. The violence in families and within individuals similarly ends when the other stops being perceived as Other.[6]

Darryl's parents had tried admonishing their son to treat the ducklings with respect, but focusing his attention on his inappropriate behavior hadn't worked. You can't force a connection to someone or something else, but you *can* invite it. By naming the ducklings and giving them imagined histories, the parents were categorizing them, outside of Darryl's awareness, as proper-named-beings-about-whom-stories-are-told, thereby connecting the birds to the people (as well, perhaps, the storybook characters) with whom he felt a special affinity or connection. This recontextualization[7] of the ducklings erased the self/Other distinction that had made the killings possible in the first place.

A similar classification process went on with Robert. Every time he made a choice between the alternatives offered to him, he accepted, outside of his awareness, the category created by the juxtaposition of the possibilities. When he decided the burglar was a he, not a she, he accepted that the shadowy presence was a gendered person (as opposed to, say, a ghost); when he decided the guy was short, rather than tall, he further accepted that he was embodied; and each of his subsequent choices—color of hair, eyes, and clothes—vivified the idea that this male person had identifiable features. Let me say it again, slightly differently: The act of choosing between or among the members of a category—separating *this* from *that*—automatically connects the distinct items, but the connection isn't noticed or perceived, so the existence of the category is affirmed on the outskirts of conscious awareness.

Bobby, Jimmy, Billy, Joey, Tommy, Scotty, Freddy, and Nicky are hanging out together. If you close your eyes and imagine what they look like, what do you see? I bet you get a picture in your mind of a bunch of young boys. Why? Our tradition in English of adding "ie" or "y" to many children's names has created a link between them, an unnamed category that evokes a sense of youth and naivete.[8] This is what I had in mind when I asked the therapists to wonder with Robert and his family whether the burglar's nickname was Rick, Ricky, or Richie. It was a context-setting way of making Richard younger, less threatening. Once the fear was embodied and comfortably named—both in Robert's imagination and in the pictures he drew—he could connect to it as an integral part of the family and as a resource for a variety of situations.

When a category or context is named, it is isolated as an object of scrutiny and can thus more easily be negated, either purposefully or out of a sense of hopelessness:

"Could you please allow us to bring this one box into the hall?"
"No, the hall is closed. You'll have to come back tomorrow."

"Darryl, why don't you treat the ducks as if they were your friends?
"No!" (snap)

"Robert, you don't know what this person you're afraid of looks like. Why not just try for a minute to get a picture in your head? Is that possible?
"No. I don't see anything. I can't."

By thinking categorically, you can prevent such knee-jerk rejections of potentially helpful ideas by establishing tacit connections—non-negation-prone contexts for therapeutic change.

## Think like a Novelist or Jazz Musician

Every time we walk into the therapy room, our clients confront us with impossible situations and painful conundrums. No wonder, then, that so many of us retreat to the seeming safety of some form of recipe-focused therapy. Faced with the frightening uncertainty of not knowing in advance how to help, we grasp for the comfortable certainty of an algorithm—a step-by-step formula that tells you what you should do and when and how you should do it.

Trouble is, if you're following a pre-established course of action, you'll be more in tune with it than with your clients. To stay in relationship with *them,* you have to be prepared and willing to work moment by moment, responding to the unique unfolding particularities of each person and situation. If you commit to extemporaneous discovery, you'll decide where to go *next* based on how your clients are responding *now* to what you *just said.* Such a welcoming of uncertainty establishes the necessary conditions for you and your clients to experience the same kind of creative immediacy enjoyed by novelists and jazz musicians.

Ursula K. LeGuin (in Coventry, 1996) once described the process of writing fiction in terms that bear directly on the practice of therapy:

> When I'm trying to control the story and make it do something, it doesn't work. When I quit trying, when I let the story tell me what it is, I get to a whole deeper level in my writing. Letting your work do itself this way requires, of course, an extremely intense, alert attitude. It's not passive; it's actively passive, passively active. (p. 42)

You can similarly choose to adopt an intense, alert attitude and let your work with your clients unfold in an actively passive, passively active way, not trying to control the particulars of their experience, and not attempting to dictate in advance what will or should happen.

I'm not suggesting you should abandon or ignore a guiding set of therapeutic principles or practices. After all, as Le Guin or any jazz musician could tell you, freedom in the absence of form is nothing but chaos. Spontaneous creativity involves the discovery of freedom *within* form. And besides, most of the best writers and jazz musicians are masters of both technique *and* theory. The trick is not letting your ideas or your approach get between you and your clients or between you and their problem.

Jazz, more than any other art form, invites and demands in-the-moment explorations of rule-bound freedom. Working within established musical parameters—modes, chord changes, melodic color tones, and time signatures—bona fide jazz musicians (not the perpetrators of the overproduced, synthesizer-enhanced, easy-listening syrup that is often marketed as "smooth jazz") devote themselves to ongoing, challenging experimentation. But to pull it off, they need to stay in continual conversation with each other; only then can they achieve the high-wire exhilaration of improvisational inter-play.

To work most effectively, we, too, must commit ourselves to collaborative spontaneity. I know of at least two hypnotherapists who tell their clients straight off to close their eyes, so they can read them a canned induction before moving on to one or more canned "thera-peutic" metaphors or stories. And I know several brief therapists who ask the same set of canned questions in the same stereotyped way in the same order at about the same time in the session, regardless of who's sitting in front of them. How deadening!

Guided, but not restricted, by your model-specific parameters, you can discover on the fly where you and your clients are heading and how you and they are getting there. This openness to not-quite-yet-knowing, this willingness and ability to continually adapt yourself to ever shifting contingencies and opportunities—this is the creative edge of novel-writing, jazz, *and* therapy.

For a year prior to first coming to see me, Brent, a twenty-five-year-old emergency-room nurse, had been waking up at night full of terror and dread, without knowing why. Sometimes as often as two or three times a night, he'd suddenly sit up in bed, his palms sweating, his heart racing, his breathing labored. He never woke with a mem-ory of dreaming, but rather with the unshakable feeling that an in-truder had entered his house. His sense of this was at times so real that his girlfriend, with whom he lived, couldn't talk him out of it, and he'd call 911. The police had been sympathetic the first time they were dispatched, but they'd since responded too many times to what they'd come to regard as crank calls, and they weren't pleased.

Brent was concerned about the police, but mostly he wanted to be able to sleep soundly and to stop feeling so afraid all the time. He was unhappy in his relationship with his girlfriend, but he was so scared to live alone that he couldn't bring himself to end it. In the preceding few years, he'd had to cope with the deaths of six family members, including two who'd passed away in his presence—his father, of liver disease, and his grandmother, of a heart attack. Brent couldn't think of his dad without shuddering at how cold and dead his hand had felt in the last moments of his life. And he couldn't think of his grandmother without seeing her face and body beneath him as he had performed the CPR that failed to save her. Despite his belief in an afterlife, and despite his not being troubled by the frequent deaths of his patients at the hospital, Brent was consumed by his kinesthetic and imagistic memories of his loved ones' dying. Terrified that some other family member might need his help in a medical emergency, he was avoiding family gatherings and refusing to visit his frail grandfather.

Brent had been seeing a therapist on and off since his dad had died, and she, recognizing that his fears and nightmares were getting in the way of his resolving his relationship with his girlfriend and relating comfortably with his family, had recommended that he come to see me for hypnosis. I anticipated working with him three to five times, but we ended up needing to meet only twice. His therapist joined us for our initial appointment but couldn't make it to the second.

I ended our first session, which I'd devoted to gathering information, by offering a different perspective on Brent's last contacts with his father and grandmother: "If I'd been your dad," I said, "I'd have been so grateful to be sent on my way with the help of your warm, strong hands—my hand enveloped in the warmth of yours. And if I'd been your grandmother, beyond pain, leaving this world, leaving my body, I'd have been so grateful to be sent on my way with your breath—my lungs filled with your spirit." I suggested that the next time someone was standing over him in a dream, he might consider helping them on their way by reaching out to or breathing into them.

When Brent arrived the following week, I likened hypnosis to what happened to him when he water skied—losing track of time, feeling "in the zone" with his skis and the tow rope and the boat's wake, and so on. I suggested that just as he relied on his body to think for itself as he carved through the water, just as his feet coordinated with his hands, and just as his hands coordinated with his legs and arms, so, too, he could allow his eyes to coordinate with other parts of his body, deciding on their own when they wanted to close.

I'd only just begun inviting Brent into the possibility of hypnosis—into concordance with himself—when he let me know that he was already ahead of me.

BRENT: Has it already started? My eyes are wanting to close and it feels funny.

I caught up as fast as I could.

DOUGLAS: Yes, it has already started. So you might as well just let your eyes do as they wish. [pause] And as they close, [pause] right, I wonder how that funny feeling will continue or change or even intensify in some way.

I juxtaposed these alternatives—continuity, change, intensification—to introduce the implicit expectation that *something,* as yet unknown, would happen to the feeling. And something did. I guess Brent found the funny feeling funny, for he started to laugh. And then he found his laughter laughable, which produced still more hilarity. I commented on how the vibration from his laughter rippled all through him, just like the vibration from his skis on the water could be felt through his entire body, and I told him about clients I'd had who'd laughed themselves *all* the way into trance. As I continued to talk about vibrations, his laughter gradually subsided. Just as it died down, someone outside started a car.

D: This is the way sound works, too, of course—through vibrations. The sound waves of that car travel from outside,

I didn't know yet where the theme of "vibrations" would take us, but the starting of the car presented an opportunity to continue playing with it, so I grabbed and ran with it.

B: I hear the car.

D: through the window, yes, through the air, and into your ear, vibrating your ear drum, which causes those three bones in your ear to vibrate, and the vibrations of the smallest one travel through the liquid in your inner ear and get all those tiny hair follicles vibrating, and they convert the vibrations to electrical signals, which then travel to your brain along your auditory nerve. That's how sound information gets transported, through vibration.

B: My fingers feel tingly.

I hadn't requested or anticipated Brent's continuing to give me a blow-by-blow account of what he was noticing, but if he was going to be good enough to provide it, I was certainly going to pay attention and improvise off of it.

D: Excellent. So let's see how the tingling changes. The sensation itself might change in some way or it may move to a different location in your body, or it may do both.

By juxtaposing these different possibilities, I was able to reinvoke the unnamed assumption, the contextualizing idea, that transformation was expectable and inevitable.

B: It's tingling in my shoulders. Not a bad tingling.

D: Great. Can the tingling get stronger?

B: Yes.

D: Would it be okay with you if it did?

B: Yes.

D: Okay, so go ahead a let it increase in strength.

This phrasing of the suggestion—rather than, for example, " . . . go ahead and increase its strength"—helped create the implication that the change was going to come from the tingling itself, not from "Brent." Acting with a mind of its own, the tingling could then surprise him. What better way to introduce the possibility of relational freedom and spontaneous change?

D: And the vibrations from that can travel to your inner ear, where you might even be able to identify them, just as if they were from a sound.

B: Pain.

D: Yes, pain. Would it be all right for that to continue for a while?

B: Yeah.

D: So let it continue, and let's see how it evolves, see how it will change.

B: Confusion.

D: Can you describe the confusion?

B: So black.

We were playing off each other here, each of us responding spontaneously to what the other was offering. I figured that if the tingling could take some kind of tangible form, it might be easier for us to work with it, but I had no preset ideas about what the form might or should be.

D: Isn't it interesting that we don't see objects per se? We see only the result of light absorbed by the object and light reflected from it. As you look at the blackness, allowing your eyes to adjust to what's absorbed and what's reflected, you may begin to see its outline, or its shape, or its pattern, or something of the sort.

Notice the tacit-category-defining options. If Brent used them to guide his search, he'd be accepting the assumption that there was indeed an *object* there to be seen. I expected his peering at the blackness to result in his discerning *something,* but I was surprised by what the object turned out to be.

B: [scowls and pauses] I see my dad.

D: Does he see you?

If the dad he was seeing was stone-cold inert, possibilities for interaction (and thus change) would be limited. My question implied that his dad had the *capacity* to see Brent, even if he wasn't presently noticing him. If his dad could scare up some personal agency, more improvisational surprises were possible.

B: I don't think so.

D: Would it be okay for you to move a little closer to him?

Brent neither nodded nor verbally acknowledged my question, so I figured I was probably moving too fast. I wanted to facilitate, not push, the possibility for interaction—connections need to be invited, not forced.

D: Or can you see well enough from here?
B: Here.
D: What do you notice?
B: His face.
D: Can you describe it?
B: He's got his gray hair.
D: His eyes?

Okay, so I didn't slow down for long. I wasn't requesting that Brent get closer to his dad, but I was asking questions that tacitly invited him to do so. He wouldn't be able to see his dad's eyes unless he was relatively close.

B: Yellow.
D: Anything else?
B: His mouth is closed.
D: Do you have any sense if he were to begin talking that you'd be able to catch what he said?

My question about proximity contains a gentle suggestion about the possibility for a conversation.

B: Don't know.
D: What about his body?
B: He's wearing a green jumpsuit.
D: What do you suppose he's wearing that for?

For a jazz improvisation to work, the musicians must always be listening closely to one another, so they can adjust what they're playing to fit with what they're hearing. The same is true for therapists. The more intimate your understanding of your clients' experience, the better able you'll be to quickly adapt to what's happening.

B: Because he's cold.
D: Socks and shoes?

B: Just socks.

D: Has he changed since the last time you saw him?

B: He's just lying there.

D: Do you have a sense of what he needs?

B: To feel better.

D: Can he tell yet that you're here?

My *yet* was Ericksonian insurance against Brent's answering the question with a *no*—it created a context for a probable shift in the current state of affairs. His dad may not have been able to sense Brent's presence, but my *yet* kept alive the possibility that this not-sensing could change at any moment.

B: Sometimes his eyes open, sometimes they don't.

He gave me an ambiguous answer (the father's open eyes might not have been taking in any information), so I looked for another way to inspire interaction.

D: Do you know yet how to help him feel better?

"Do you know *yet?*"—more insurance.

B: I don't think I can.

D: Your and his understanding of what he needs from you could be quite different.

I wanted to leave open the possibility that, even though Brent might think he couldn't help, his dad might know how he could.

D: Is it okay for you to move a little closer?

He hadn't grabbed hold of any of the "why-don't-you-interact-with-him?" options I'd been offering, so I tried reintroducing my first idea.

B: Yes.

D: So go ahead and do that and notice what happens with your dad when you do.

My phrasing strongly suggested that *something* would happen when he moved closer, but I left it up to Brent to discover what it would be.[9]

B:  He sat up.
D:  Yeah.

Encouraged by the dad's dramatic response, I took the opportunity to connect it to another to-be-discovered change.

D:  Interesting that he only did that when you got physically closer to him. Look more closely in his face and see what you didn't see before.
B:  He looks scared.
D:  So now you see fear, you know what he needs. Look inside your body for inspiration and see what you can do. You don't need to do it yet, just discover what it is. As you listen to yourself, what comes to mind?

Brent stayed silent, so I tried a new tack.

D:  You might try telling him it's okay and see how he reacts.
B:  He still looks confused.
D:  Go inside again and look for another idea—you don't have to be right the first time. Let me know when something comes to mind.
B:  Don't know.

The Christmas when our son Eric was two and a half, our friend William came over to help us trim our tree. As Eric hung an ornament on one of the branches, William complimented him on the *perfection* of his placement. An instant later, Eric yanked the decoration off and rehung it a few branches over. Without pausing for a breath, William continued, "But of course that *too* is an ideal location." I did my best to match William's swift grace as I responded to Brent's comment.

D:  No reason you should. So *discover* it by asking your dad and letting him tell you.
B:  My toes are tingling.

I figured the tingling had something to do with my earlier suggestion that he look inside his body for inspiration. I just hadn't given his body the necessary time to develop something.

D: Wonderful. Listen to that vibration with your inner ear and when you hear what that tingling is saying now, let me know. What is that tingling signaling?

If jazz musicians can return to earlier established themes, why not us?

B: Lots of things. Too many of them.
D: See if you can tease them apart.

Brent started describing his grandmother's fighting with his girlfriend; I considered this a digression, so I brought the focus back to his father. My next few contributions to the interchange went nowhere, but then we started cooking, again:

D: You saw that he sat up when you got closer before. Would getting still closer to him be okay with you?
B: Yes.
D: Okay, so do that, and see what happens in his face.
B: He's crying.
D: Yes. . . . He's able to cry, now.

I framed the dad's crying as a step forward, a development arising from Brent's getting closer to him.

D: Do you know yet how to help him?
B: He wants to hug me.
D: Yes, he does.

As I spoke, he exhaled forcefully and appeared to be experiencing the hug.

D: [long pause] What's happening?
B: He's still hugging me.
D: Can you hug him back?
B: [nods slightly]

Ever remember being unilaterally hugged by someone? It felt like the other person was violating your space, right? I figured the embrace had more potential to be therapeutic if Brent could experience himself actively participating in it, rather than being subjected to it. He'd been recoiling from his fear for a long time—this was a chance to reach out and connect with it, to become of one mind with it.

D: Because that *is* what he needs, isn't it?

A few seconds after I said this, Brent started coughing violently, and he continued, on and off, for the next couple of minutes. By the time he was finished, his eyes, which had opened, were watery from the exertion. He wasn't focusing on anything in the room, though, so I waited until his eyelids had closed again before checking in with him.

D: And now what's happening?
B: He's just looking.
D: Where?
B: At me.

As I had with the hugging, I presumed that Brent would feel like a helpless victim if his connection with his dad wasn't mutual. Being stared at is unnerving; actively looking into someone's eyes creates intimacy.

D: Can you meet his gaze? Allow him to look in your eyes? Allow yourself to look in his eyes?

He cried quietly for a few minutes, which appeared to relax him.

D: That's right.

I waited several more minutes before again asking about his experience.

D: What's happening?
B: He told me he's proud of me.
D: Ahhh. You'll want to protect that, I'm sure, in a very special place—somewhere you can always return to and have access to.

I suggested the possibility of amnesia and then invited him to reorient to the room. He was surprised when he looked at his watch and when he noticed his wet cheeks.

B:  I guess I cried?

This session felt to me like an improvisational duet. Staying in close contact, Brent and I were each able to respond with immediacy to what, at the moment, the other was offering. My questions and suggestions were guided by ideas about connecting with problems and so on, but I wasn't following a step-by-step recipe for achieving "positive results." I was following *him*.[10]

A few months later, Brent's therapist e-mailed me with an update:

> Today, the client I had referred to you came in to figure out some things regarding his girlfriend. He said that since his last meeting with you, he hasn't been having those dreams that would wake him up, and, over the holiday, he had no difficulty being with his family. He is now comfortable sleeping alone and being alone. He believes his fears prevented him from truly evaluating his feelings for his girlfriend . . . I detected a huge difference in his talk.

Freed from his fear and foreboding, Brent ended his relationship with his girlfriend. He later started a relationship with someone new and, a year and a half later, married her.

## Date, but Never Marry, Your Ideas

Even if you're adept at offering new ideas to clients, sometimes you'll find yourself with a notion that makes perfect sense to you but seems like perfect nonsense to them, or one that makes sense to both of you but ends up not helping. I never give up on an idea immediately, at least not one I'm pretty sure could potentially make a difference in my clients' lives. But clients are the final arbiters, so I always value my relationship with them over my relationship with a frame or a direction that isn't working for them. I'd like to tell you two stories—the first illustrates the importance of not abandoning a good idea too quickly; the second, of not holding onto a good (but unhelpful) idea too tightly or too long.

When Kristin, one of my students, came back behind the one-way mirror for a mid-session consultation, she started off the conversation with an apology. A few minutes earlier, while empathizing with her Chilean client, Maria, Kristin had asked her whether she felt "cursed" by a comment her ex-husband had made the last time he'd seen her. Maria had implied as much in the story she'd told us, but the word itself wasn't hers, and Kristin was worried that she'd inadvertently risked making Maria's situation worse. What if her client felt over-whelmed by having to carry the extra burden of a curse on top of everything else she was having to contend with?

I generally encourage my students not to venture too far beyond the vocabulary and language style of their clients, but this situation struck me as unique. Kristin had, to my ear, found the *perfect* frame to capture the tenor and long-term consequences of what the ex had said. When Maria and her then husband had parted three years earlier, he had proclaimed that she was going to remain alone for the rest of her life and that no one would love her for *her*—only for the sex she could provide. Unable to forget his angry declaration, and blaming herself for the failure of two subsequent relationships, Maria had expected us to confirm that she was as bad and hopeless as her ex had claimed.

Kristin, the team, and I suspected that Maria was suffering not from some character defect, but from a self-fulfilling prophecy. Anticipating that her relationships would fail, she seemed to have acted in ways that furthered their demise. We had a hunch that if she could bring herself to question the validity of her self-blaming and negative expectations, she'd be freed up to act differently the next time she met a potential partner. Kristin's frame, then, seemed ideal, for, if accepted, it would allow Maria to lay the blame for her nega-tive experiences on the curse rather than on herself. Therapy could then focus on the simple task of removing the curse and facilitate Maria's learning how to trust herself.

Only one problem: When Kristin introduced the idea of her having been cursed, Maria laughingly dismissed it. Respectful and cau-tious—to my taste, too cautious—Kristin let it drop and moved on. But I wasn't ready to give up so easily, so I called in (on the telephone connecting the observation and therapy rooms) and asked Kristin to tell Maria that because she'd never stopped believing what her hus-band had said to her, the team still believed she'd been cursed. Maria told Kristin that she did indeed believe her ex's words, but she didn't consider his words to have been a curse. Fortunately, Kristin had the presence of mind to ask Maria how she could tell the difference.

During the course of their subsequent conversation, Kristin reiterated her understanding of Maria's situation, and Maria for the first time began to take her seriously. In concluding the session, Kristin told her that she and the team knew several ways to deal with curses and that, if she thought it'd be helpful, we'd be happy to share them with her the following week.

The next appointment turned out to be Maria's last, as she was planning to leave soon for an extended trip to Chile. She began the session by telling Kristin that she now thought maybe she *had* been cursed, but she also believed she had something wrong inside her. I called in and asked Kristin to tell her that the most difficult curses are those that make you believe there is something wrong inside when the only problem is the curse itself. Maria replied that her father had inadvertently participated in invoking and maintaining the curse by sending her monthly letters from Chile, urging her not to trust men. She planned to see him and talk to him about the curse when she returned home, but she thought that she herself would need to be the one to lift it. We suggested that the trip to Chile might be an ideal time to initiate such a process, and Kristin asked Maria to contact her when she returned.

Two months later, Maria called and said that the curse was no longer a problem. While in Chile, she had spoken to her father, who had acknowledged the curse-like nature of her exhusband's proclamation. By virtue of her father's understanding, she said, the curse had been lifted, and her ex's words had lost their power to influence her.

Kristin learned that you can respect your clients *and* hold onto a frame they initially reject. If you have an idea—or even just a hunch—that seems to fit their experience, and if it has the potential to change their relationship to their problem, your clients deserve a chance to give it a chance. You neither want to abandon a frame too readily nor grip it too tenaciously.

Dierdre, a young English woman in the States on business, had been blessed with a fair complexion and a flair for noticing unintended double entendres. The combination had not been a happy one. During conversations with friends, coworkers, and family members, she couldn't help herself from latching onto words that could be interpreted—usually out of context—as oblique references to something sexual. The thought would produce a blush and then, afraid that the other person would clue into what had triggered her reaction (and conclude she had "a filthy mind"), she'd redden still more.

Dierdre had what she described as a healthy, open attitude about sex, so she couldn't understand why she automatically found sexual significance in "innocent" words and why her body insisted on responding to them so dramatically. A previous therapist in England had introduced thought-stopping (and other) techniques, but nothing had worked. "By the time I'd reach over to snap the elastic on my wrist," Dierdre explained, "the blush had already started." She'd tried her best to keep her thinking process in check, but, predictably, this had only exacerbated the situation.

Rather than intervene by trying to help her better control her thoughts and her body, I *intra*vened by looking for a way she could allow her natural proclivities to take her someplace new. I pointed out that she had a quick-witted, punning mind, an irrepressible, mischievous sense of humor, and a healthy body that knew how to move blood to different places in response to cues from her environment. In regular social situations, sexual innuendos, even (or perhaps especially) when unintentional, invited her blood to move north, producing a blush. But in intimate situations, such as when she and her boyfriend were in the mood for making love, such innuendos invited her blood to move *south,* producing the swelling of her vulva and the lubrication of her vagina.

I clarified that we couldn't change her complexion or the ability of her face to show embarrassment. "But we might be able to use hypnosis," I suggested, "to help your body learn, in non-intimate social situations, to send blood south instead of north. You have stressed the gravity of your predicament, so we might as well let gravity help out. If your blood's going to move in response to your ability to hear sexual double meanings, it might as well move to the parts of your body that most directly relate to the words themselves. Why shouldn't your blood move down to your genitals, rather than up to your face?"

I made sure that Dierdre would be comfortable becoming "privately sexually aroused" when she heard double entendres and that she was confident her ability to get turned on would be noticeable to no one but herself. I also asked her permission to talk to her during hypnosis in such a way that she could allow her body to listen to my words and send her blood south.[11] She was fine with the idea, so we proceeded in this direction for a few sessions. I purposefully used every innuendo I could think of, interspersing them with suggestions for arousal and for going into social situations *anticipating* cues for southward blood flow, for swelling and lubricating.

Dierdre's career took her back to England at this point, and I didn't hear from her for six months. One day she called to say she was flying in for a week of business meetings. The blushing had improved "somewhat"—she no longer entered conversations with the same degree of anticipation and anxiety—but she'd also had some "setbacks," so she wanted to schedule a few more hypnosis sessions. She said that although she understood the rationale for the direction of the previous sessions, she didn't really think they'd worked.

Searching for another way of proceeding, I paid more attention to a detail that I'd previously heard but not highlighted. Dierdre's sexual antennae would go up if, for example, her boss stressed the necessity of keeping *abreast* of shifts in the market or if a coworker asked her *to come* to lunch. Although such phrases were enough to get a little blood moving upward, the flood came when she worried about the other person figuring out the *pattern* of her blushing and concluding that she was some kind of pervert. It made sense, then, that she wouldn't have to blush so much if she could only blush *more*—often enough, at least, to ensure no one would be able to crack the code.

If her reddening only happened in response to words easily recognizable as potential sexual puns—*head, finger, lips, penetration, fantasy, suck,* and so on—people might quite easily connect Dierdre's blushing to the use of the words in a conversation. But such sleuthing would be impossible if she increased the sensitivity of her double-entendre radar to include totally innocent sounding, mundane words. If she could redden at *abreast* or *come,* why not at *but?* All she needed to do was add an automatic *t* to the end of it when she heard it, and she could be on her way. And this wasn't the only word with promising automatic titillation possibilities. Inviting her into concordance, I suggested she let her quick-witted mind supply a letter here or a letter there, and maybe the odd word here or there, thereby creating an *orgy* of meaning in almost every sentence. Quick as a blush, she could add an *out* when she heard someone say *in,* add an *s* to the word *as,* put a *t* in front of the word *it,* or attach a *gasm* to *or.* Imagine what she could manage to hear sitting across from some American at lunch who happened to say, "But what's it like working in England? Is it just me or is it as dreary as I've heard?":"*Butt* what's *tit* like working *in and out* England? Is *tit* just me *orgasm* is it *ass* dreary *ass* I've heard?" And if this didn't keep her busy enough, she could allow her ear to catch every word starting with the letter *f* and let each one bring to mind the sound and image of *the f*-word.

Two months after Dierdre returned to England, we talked on the phone, and she told me things were better. Whenever she started to anticipate hearing double entendres, she said, she'd "destroy the pattern" by trying to blush as much and as often as possible. As a result, her blushing hadn't "been that bad" and, when it did happen, she would "just accept" it as part of who she was. I still like the quirky logic of the first approach we tried, but not enough to have chosen it over my client.

## *Inviting Change*

In the process of talking about how to orient to change, I've said quite a bit about how to help implement it. I'd like now like to focus more directly on the specifics of getting things moving—on how to invite, recognize, nurture, and midwife nascent changes as they occur within and between sessions.

### Invite Clients to Connect with Their Problem

To get your and your clients' therapeutic creativity sparking, you and they need to feel comfortable and safe not only with each other (see Chapters 3 and 4), but also with their problem. As long you and/or they are trying to protect yourselves *from* whatever it is they're struggling against—rage, pain, panic, depression, suicidal or paranoid ideation, self-destructive urges and behaviors, and so on—your efforts will be restricted to separative strategies, involving attempts at either eradication or control.

The word *control* comes from the Latin *contra* against and *rotulus* roll: to turn against. You may find it necessary at times to turn against a symptom, particularly if you or your clients are in danger. But the short-term benefit of such a divisive action can produce a long-term exacerbation of the situation. Anytime you attempt to create safety for you or your clients by protecting them from what they hate or fear, you make it impossible for them to relax into trusting themselves. If their safety depends on constant vigilance, what happens when they lose focus or become bored, discouraged, or exhausted? A forced separation creates a separated connection, which keeps the symptom alive and well.

The alternative is to foster a non-forced connection between your clients and whatever's grabbing them around the throat, resulting in, or at least making possible, a connected separation, gap of insignificance. When the relationship transforms, so does the throat-grabber.

Therapists familiar with symptom prescription (a species of paradoxical intervention) have sometimes asked me whether this is what I'm up to when I'm inviting clients to hang out with their symptom in a new way, suggesting they get curious about it, protect time for it, honor it, experiment with it, learn from it. I tell them they might make sense of my work this way, but I don't. Let me tell you why.

Strategic (Haley, 1984; Madanes, 1984) and MRI (Watzlawick, Weakland, & Fisch, 1974) therapists, as well as the original Milan team (Selvini Palazzoli, Boscolo, Cecchin, & Prata, 1978), highlight the benefits of placing clients in a "therapeutic paradox," encouraging them to purposefully perform (or have, or maintain) their symptom. If the clients rebel, refusing to "do" the problem as suggested, then they are no longer held captive by it. And if, in contrast, they follow the therapist's instructions and manage to *make* the problem happen, then the symptom, no longer a spontaneous behavior with a mind of its own, becomes purposeful, and the clients are no longer its passive victims.

Paradoxical interventions are generally thought of as "powerful," for they can produce dramatic effects in short periods of time. But if you approach clients with the intent of "paradoxing" them out of their problem, you position yourself as an outsider. I prefer to use metaphoric thinking to get *inside* the logic and lived complexity of their experience, where I can invent and develop *intra*ventions— possibilities for change that evolve from *within* the relationship between the clients and their problem.

The idea behind all intraventions, regardless of their idiosyncratic particulars, is to provide clients an opportunity to connect with their problem and/or with something else. An atmosphere of "invitation" is central to the process. You can't simply demand that your clients connect with their throat-grabber, explaining (or even just implying) that their separation attempts are wrong. If you only give them a negation-based means of changing ("You need to stop trying to stop your problem—it's time to make friends with it"), all they can do is attempt to separate from their separating ("You're right—I just have to stop running away! I have to force myself turn around and face my fear!"). As a result, they'll be as entangled in knots as they were before coming to see you—or even more so.

One of the more elegant ways to invite a non-coerced connection between your clients and their problem is to encourage their curiosity about their experience. When you suggest they gather detailed information about their symptom—when it happens, when it doesn't, how fast it comes on, how long (or short) it lasts, how it spins out of control, how predictable or unpredictable it is, and so on— you'll be offering an opportunity for them to move toward something from which they've been backing away. The insider data they garner for you will give you loads of intraventive ideas for how the problem might then be tickled into changing, but sometimes their data-gathering alone will make all the difference.

Back when I was in graduate school, I and two of my colleagues (who served as a behind-the-mirror team for me)[12] saw a client, Nichola, who was worried she might be bulimic. She'd been binge-ing and vomiting for a while but only recently had become concerned enough to seek professional help. Wanting to get a sense of the seriousness of her situation so she could decide whether she needed to pursue in-depth therapy, she requested a diagnosis of her condition. I asked lots of specific questions about how, what, when, how often, and with whom she ate, as well as how, how often, when, and with whom she threw up. Some of the questions she could answer; some, she couldn't—at least not yet.

After taking a consultation break with my colleagues, I talked again with Nichola, telling her, "You've come in asking for help in determining whether you're bulimic. We don't know at this point whether you are or not, so we need to investigate it further with you.

We'd thus like to ask you to closely observe your eating and throwing up for the next week, write down whatever seems relevant, and come back in a week and tell us about it."

When Nichola came back, she told us she'd taken detailed notes and, although she wasn't sure, she thought perhaps, for whatever reason, she'd thrown up less this last week than she had during previous weeks. She and I explored her experience in depth, and then I went back behind the mirror for a consult. My colleagues and I decided that, since she was in search of a diagnosis, we'd be wise to give her one, but something more hopeful than "bulimia." I went back in the room and said, "We can't be certain, but what we're thinking at this point is that you probably aren't suffering from bulimia; we think, actually, you're suffering from *quasi-bulimia*." I explained that quasi-bulimia is similar to bulimia, but that it differs in precipitating factors and prognosis. "But since we can't be certain," I went on, "we'd like you to collect some further information for us, and we'll firm up our diagnosis more at the next appointment." We didn't tell her to try to do anything different about the throwing up, only to pay even closer attention to the microdynamics of her experience.

Two weeks later, Nichola came back and told us that for some strange reason she hadn't thrown up much at all since she'd last been to see us, so she didn't have as much information to give us as she'd hoped. After she and I had delved into what she *had* managed to discover, I took my consultation break and then, based on my conversations with my team, came back and announced, "We're thinking now the difficulty is not quasi-bulimia after all; rather, we suspect you're suffering from *pseudo-bulimia*." The new provisional diagnosis was, of course, even more hopeful than the last, but since we still couldn't be certain, it only made sense for Nichola to continue with her close observations. These were ostensibly serving to help us come up with the "proper" diagnosis, but, of course, they were also transforming her relationship to eating and throwing up.

When Nichola came back for what turned out to be her last appointment, she told me she hadn't thrown up at all since our previous session. She had, though, taken notes about her eating, so we went over those in great detail before I again conferred with my colleagues. When I came back in from my break, I told her that we now recognized she wasn't pseudo-bulimic after all. "Rather," I said, "we recognize, as you do, that you sometimes have an issue with eating." Much relieved, Nichola decided that she didn't require therapy for this, and she left—not a bulimic, not a quasi-bulimic, not even a pseudo-bulimic. She sometimes had an issue with food.

## Invite Clients to Connect to Something Else

By connecting with a problem from which you've been trying to separate, you create the possibility of your separated connection transforming into a connected separation, of your throwing-away turning into a letting-go. Something similar happens when, instead of focusing your efforts on separating from the problem, you find yourself connecting to something else, instead. The more captivating or interesting this something else is, the less important, the less noticeable, the problem becomes.

A few years ago, my friend Sandra Roscoe, an expert in hypnosis and meditation, needed to get a biopsy of some suspicious cysts, and she asked me for any ideas I might have to help her ready herself for the procedure. She had been trying to prepare on her own, using both her daily meditation practice and self-hypnosis, but she was having trouble. Every time she sat down to "be" with the impending biopsy and the flurry of concerns, thoughts, and images that were coming to her, she felt pulled to take her dog for a walk, to put together a lecture for one of the classes she was teaching, to busy herself in the kitchen, and so on. With the appointment fast approaching, she was worried that she wouldn't be properly prepared.

I knew from experience that Sandra was wonderfully adept at immersing herself in her experience and, as a result, losing track of other stuff around her. I noted that since her "distractability" wasn't itself a problem—she was taking the situation seriously, she'd made an appointment with her doctor as soon as she'd noticed the cysts, and she had every intention of following through with the biopsy—she might as well respect it as a perfectly acceptable means of responding to the situation. Instead of trying so hard to "be" with the cysts and her fear that they might be cancerous—that is, instead of trying to connect with them—why not allow herself get drawn into the pleasures and demands of her busy and productive life?

Sandra told me that, when she'd had dental work done, she'd avoided the use of anesthesia by cycling through what she called three different "stations of awareness." She'd get curious about the sensations on the bottom of one of her feet, then move to noticing the weight of the instruments on her chest, and then open herself to noticing the variety of sounds in the room. As she'd go around and around, successively touching base with whatever was going on at each station, she'd lose track of the sensations in her mouth.

We agreed that such cycling would undoubtedly prove helpful during her biopsy, too. It made sense for Sandra to keep the foot and room-sound stations, but what, she wondered, should she use for the third? Given that new stuff kept popping into her head every time she sat down to focus her attention, I wondered whether she might want to build this in as an essential element of her self-hypnotic experience. Why not create a station of unpredictability? She could cycle from her foot to the room sounds to, say, a blank screen of awareness, knowing that every time she arrived at this screen, something new and surprising would be waiting there for her: an image of her husband building something, the sense of her home in North Carolina, the sound and feel of her dog barking and jumping up on her, the sight of her favorite five-year-old (my son) smiling at her, and so on. Appreciating the opportunity this would afford for creative discovery, she looked forward to giving it a try.

As the doctor started examining her, Sandra cycled her awareness around the three stations. Her foot felt comfortable, the sounds in the room, she told me later, were "very very far away," and every time she came back to her place of surprise, she was astonished and delighted by what she found there. By connecting to the movement of her mind and the surprises it held in store, she lost track of what the doctor and nurses were up to. Only when she heard them cheering did she reorient to the room and discover the happy news: Since the cysts were all able to be aspirated, no biopsy was necessary, after all.

## Look for the Fit, Rather than the Function, of Symptoms

Strategic therapists commonly look for how symptoms serve positive purposes in their clients' lives—how a daughter's depression keeps her parents from following through with a threatened divorce, how a husband's weight gain keeps his wife's jealousy in check, how vociferous arguments keep passion alive in an otherwise stale marriage.

Adopting such an approach will effectively keep you from trying to help your clients get rid of their symptom. After all, you aren't going to try to eradicate something you're claiming to be functionally necessary for the balance of their current state of affairs. But once you've committed yourself to singing the praises of the symptom, you've limited your freedom for subsequent sessions.[13]

A therapist I know was seeing a client who couldn't stop thinking about one of her former boyfriends. Several months after breaking up with him, she still couldn't keep her mind on her work; she was making daily trips to his neighborhood, hoping for a glimpse of him and his new lover; and she was sprinkling his name into every conversation she had with her girlfriends. The therapist pointed out that her obsession was protective of her, as it was helping to ensure that she didn't prematurely go out and get into another bad relationship. The woman agreed, but, after several weeks of hearing the same thing, she asked an excellent question: "Yeah, okay, but now what?"

Rather than looking for the function of a symptom, I look for its *fit*—how it has become an integrated part of my clients' life and how the relationship between it and my clients can be invited to *dis*integrate. By attending to the strands of habit and expectation that have kept the symptom knotted in place, I keep its context always in mind. But I don't adopt the position that my clients won't be able to live without it, and I'm not interested in trying to get them to prove me wrong. Instead, I look for how the strands can be unknotted, for how a change in the relationship to the symptom can be accompanied, or even initiated, by a change in one or more other relationships.

I once consulted on a case involving a seven-year-old girl— Isadora—whose nightmares scared her so much that she was afraid to go to bed at night. She couldn't fall asleep unless her light was left on, and when she'd jolt awake at night in the middle of one of the dreams, she'd need one of her parents to help her stop crying and settle back down—a process that could take up to an hour. Exhausted and frustrated, her parents disagreed on the best course of action to improve the situation. They'd already ruled out the possibility that she was being mistreated at school or somehow being abused, and no friends or extended family members had recently died or been seriously ill. They were thus at a loss for why the nightmares would be so intense and unrelenting.

The therapist, Sean, believed that the daughter's problem was serving a positive function in the family, helping to distract the parents from an as-yet-unearthed marital problem. With this in mind, he had broached the possibility of the couple's coming in alone to talk about their marriage, but they had balked.[14] Not sure of where to go next, he asked me to observe the case from behind a one-way mirror and to offer any suggestions I might have for how he and the family could get beyond their impasse.

I agreed, and, after watching for a while, I called into Sean with an idea. Reasoning that Isadora's nightmares wouldn't be so vivid if she didn't possess a remarkable imagination, I thought it worthwhile to assess the degree of her artistic ability. I thus suggested that Sean begin testing her creative potential.

Could she close her eyes and imagine a red dot?

Yes, as it turned out, she could.

Could she expand the red dot into a red square?

Yes.

Excellent. Could she turn the square into a triangle?

No.

Of course not. Who could do that? Okay, could she shrink the square back to a dot?

Yup.

And then expand the dot into a triangle?

Uh huh.

And back to a dot?

Yup.

And turn the red dot into a blue dot?

Yes.

And expand the blue dot into a blue circle?

Yes!

Isadora demonstrated excellent imaginative skills, beyond what her mom and dad would have guessed.

We decided, based on these initial results, that we needed further information, so we asked the parents to continue the assessment throughout the week. Having secured their agreement, we sent them off to a local art-supply store to purchase a box of pencil crayons and some good quality paper. Every night, they were to give Isadora ten to twenty minutes of time alone in her room, so she could draw and color the nightmare she anticipated having. When she was done, the parents were then to come into her room together, sit on her bed, and talk with her about what she'd rendered.

Isadora might, we warned, find her imagination beginning to flag after a few nights of this exercise. If this were to happen, she could always implement something she'd learned during the session. Just as closing her eyes had helped her better picture the changing size, shape, and color of the objects she'd seen in her head, so too being treated to a little darkness would probably help her more vividly imagine the night's anticipated nightmare. If she were to find herself in need of such a creative nudge, then her parents should switch off her light, leave the room for sixty seconds, come back, turn the light on again, and then give Isadora time alone to bring the necessary vitality to her artwork. If, on subsequent nights, Isadora were to again feel uninspired, her parents should increase the length of her darkness-aided imagination, sixty seconds at a time.

Just before they left the session, we asked the parents to facilitate one further evaluation of their daughter's imaginative and artistic abilities. In addition to the evening drawings of *anticipated* nightmares, we would like to see, we said, early morning sketches of any *actual* nightmares. The morning drawings, however, should be half the size of the evening ones, as this would allow us to assess not only the similarities and differences between Isadora's expectations and her experience, but also her sense of proportion. We left it up to the parents to explain to Isadora what we meant by this.

The family returned two weeks later, apologetic that Isadora had managed to complete only six sketches—four full-sized evening drawings and two half-sized morning ones. The parents, working together, had done their best to gather the information we'd requested, but they'd had trouble making it happen. On the third night of the assessment, Isadora felt bored, so they switched off her light to help inspire her imagination. It worked that and the next night, but on the fifth night, when they returned to her room to switch her light back on, they discovered that she'd fallen asleep. Hating to disturb her, they took the art supplies off her bed and tucked her in.

The same thing happened the next few nights, and, after that, they could no longer convince Isadora to bother with the drawings. Her nightmares stopped, so she no longer had anything to draw when she woke up, either.[15] We admired the quality of the pictures she'd managed to complete, noting that they did, indeed, demonstrate a marvelous artistic sensibility, but we agreed with the parents that since the nightmares had stopped and Isadora now had no problem falling asleep with the light off, further assessment of her creative abilities would be better conducted by an art, dance, drama, or music teacher.

By requesting an assessment of Isadora's artistic ability, the therapist was able to join with the parents, they were able join with each other, and everyone was able to connect with the nightmares and the darkened room. Getting disentangled from a symptom is always easier when the relational strands holding it in place are loosened.

## Work at Altering, Rather than Negating, Your Clients' Symptom[16]

As I explained in Chapter 1, whenever your clients try to negate (banish, abolish, discount) some chunk of their experience (thoughts, pain, voices, memories, emotions), they forge a divisive relationship with it—a separated connection. If they persist in and/or intensify such disjunctive efforts, the chunk will take on leechlike qualities, becoming a symptom or problem capable of frustrating any attempts (theirs or yours) at controlling or eradicating it. Recognizing this relational quality of language and mind, you'll do best to organize your therapy around *altering,* rather than *negating,* their symptom.

Carrie and Sam both agreed that Carrie was "hypervigilant" about keeping her sons safe and well, so much so that she was constantly distraught that one of them would catch a cold or sprain an ankle. At its worst, Carrie's worry was debilitating for her and restrictive for her boys, as she would constrain their activities way beyond what they and Sam thought was remotely reasonable. But despite their protestations, nothing could dissuade her from taking extra measures to keep her family safe. Nothing, indeed, could keep the severe voice in her head from whispering, "Did you do enough?"

Carrie could quiet the voice for brief periods by heeding all its admonishments and demands, but it remained ever wary, always prepared to reproach her for making the tiniest little slip. And if she mustered the temerity to reassure herself that she was doing a good job, she'd be subjected to withering criticism. Sam worked hard to reassure her of her positive qualities, and this sometimes helped, but if the voice considered her the least bit neglectful, its invectives would become unrelenting.

I invited her into concordance with herself in the last half of the second session. Carrie decided she wanted Sam to stick around, though she was initially uncomfortable with his looking at her. I suggested they both focus on the same spot in front of them, as if they were watching a movie together; this helped Carrie relax into the experience. Then, as I commented on ambient sounds, speculated about possible thoughts and sensations, and offered possible experiences, she stopped bothering to distinguish herself from me, her body, and her surroundings. Tears appeared occasionally on her cheeks. When she reoriented to the room at the end, she said that, during the time I was talking, she was seeing an image of herself at thirteen, sitting on the floor in her room next to her bed, looking at her closed door and feeling incredibly sad. Not having planned or attempted to evoke any memories, I was surprised and encouraged by the spontaneous freedom of her response. Noting that sadness is different from anxiety, I scheduled the next appointment.

When the couple returned the following week, Carrie said that she'd woken up the day after our last session feeling more peaceful and hopeful than she had in years. We talked about her sensitivity and about the interesting way emotions evolve when freed up to be themselves. After inviting her into trance and telling her a story about being at the movies with my wife, I suggested that she, too, could focus her attention on a screen in front of her, watching what happened and filling me in on the details.

CARRIE: I see my mother in my room. Her back is to me. She's angry.

Like the week before, we were back in her room, but this time she wasn't alone.

DOUGLAS: How can you tell she's angry?

Had she used past tense, I would have invited her into using present, but she was already ahead of me.

C: [pause] She just is.
D: Is it the tension in her back, the tilt of her head, her body position?

I prefer descriptions to conclusions, as they offer readier opportunities for transformation.

C: She's above me. She's big.

D: How old are you?

C: I don't know—thirteen, fourteen, maybe fifteen.

D: Are you sitting or standing?

C: I'm sitting on the floor by the bed.

D: And how can you see her anger? How can you tell?

C: In her mouth. [pause] Her mouth is angry and her eyes are disappointed.

D: And where is she?

C: In the room. I'm looking up at her.

Sitting on the floor, looking up: a vulnerable, submissive position.

D: All the way in?

C: She's partly in. She always passes by me. She's distant. She's not close. She's always disappointed in me. I can't be the way she wants me to be.

D: How is that?

C: She wants me to do things like her, do them her way. [pause] I can't do that. She's so sad. She misses me, too.

What a wonderful opening! She spoke the I words "I can't do that" with a tone of guilty defeat, but they held the potential for defiant integrity.

D: Go inside and find that voice of yours that's wise enough to know that, despite your mother's pain, her disappointment, her sadness, her anger, despite all that, it's necessary for you to do things *your* way. Go and listen to that voice, that necessary, wise voice, and tell me what it's saying.

C: [long pause] I can't find it. Her voice is so loud.

In the first session, Carrie had described trying unsuccessfully to "brush the voice away." But even if she were to manage to briefly brush it off, this would only encourage it to fight back. The key was to find a way to *alter,* not negate, it.

D: Well, it's important to be respectful of your mother's presence, so you don't want to try to shut up, to shut out what she is saying, but it *is* difficult to hear two things at the same time. [pause] So go ahead and turn down the volume of her voice so you can hear yourself think. [long pause] My mother used to come to my door and yell, "Turn that music down! I can't hear myself think!" That was good motherly advice: Turn down the volume so you can hear yourself think. So go ahead and turn down the volume of your mother's advice so you can hear yourself think. And you might as well lower the illumination on her as well, so you can see better, too. Nothing like a little subdued lighting and background music to encourage self-reflection. [long pause] Now go inside again and tell me what you can hear that wise voice saying.

C: It is saying, "I *am* smart!"

She sounded defensive. I was concerned that if the defensiveness remained, her definition of herself as smart would stay bound to her mother's accusation that she wasn't. Not wanting her positive assertion automatically invoking its negation, I looked for a way of easing the two apart, of creating a gap of insignificance.

D: Fine. What is the quality of that voice?
C: [pause] It is angry.
D: Sure, for good reason. Go ahead and take the anger out of that wise voice and listen again. [pause] Now how does it sound?

I wish I hadn't been so abrupt. Rather than trying to snatch the anger away, I should have given it the opportunity to evolve into some other emotion. Or I could have suggested that she let it increase, and as she felt it rising higher and higher, she might begin to notice it pulling another emotion into the light. And as this other emotion appeared and developed, the anger, having been so helpful, could now be free to continue on its way, out the door, through the ceiling, into the ether, or whatever. Oh well.

C: [long pause] It sounds calmer. Freer and calmer.
D: Right. And now what's happening?
C: Is it true? What if I'm wrong? I'm scared.

D: Okay, well that, too, is an important voice, so listen carefully to it, as well. And like the other voice, allow this voice to tell you its important message. Notice that, as you listen to it, respecting it, the edge can come off it. [long pause] And now how does it sound?

C: [pause] Smaller.

D: Okay, but don't let it get too small, because it is important that it has a conversation with the voice that is saying, "I am smart." So go ahead and let them converse, [pause] and tell me what happens.

The voice of fear was now her own. I made the assumption that if, instead of trying to quell it, she were to listen to and respect it, it wouldn't have to yell at her.

C: [long pause] The scared voice says, "I don't want to mess up," and the smart voice is reassuring it.

D: I have a suggestion for the smart voice.

At this point I personified the two voices—a way for me to demonstrate my respect. I talked to the smart one directly and used the pronoun *her* to refer to the scared one.

D: I wonder what would happen if you were to [pause] to reassure the scared voice in a different way. If you didn't try to settle her down. If you respected her for helping you be smart. So I wonder what might happen if you were to reassure the scared voice that you won't let her disappear, reassure her that she keeps you smart, [pause] that you'll always listen to her because she makes you smarter.

I then switched back to talking to "Carrie," rather than the "voice."

D: Go ahead and let the smart voice tell the scared voice something like that and let me know what happens.

C: [long pause] The scared voice isn't scared anymore. Just sad.

D: Okay, listen to that, and wait to see how it continues to change.

If you accept and respect your clients' nonvolitional response, not trying to negate it and building the expectancy that it will transform, *something*—Who know's what?—will happen.

C: [long pause] Now it is peace.

D: Peace. Yes. And now what?

C: Bright.

D: What sort of brightness?

C: Like the sun. Very bright.

D: Now is this just the scared voice that has become this, or?

C: No.

D: Is it possible to even identify the smart voice and the scared voice separately?

My *even* heightened the likelihood that they'd be experienced as one.

C: No.

D: [pause] Well, how appropriate that smart and scared together would be *bright*. Very bright.

I don't know whether her imagination was punning on the double meaning of bright, but even if it wasn't, I couldn't resist.

C: It is filtered now, like through trees.

D: So there are some shadows, too?

C: Yes.

D: Oh wonderful, for shadows are important, too. You always need both the brightness and some shadows, some dappled light and shadows.

My comment allowed me to offer again, this time metaphorically, the idea of embracing, rather than expelling.

D: Now put this in a safe place within you, a place that you can always return to. And your dreams at night can continue the process here. Have you found a safe place to keep this?

C: Yes. [smiles]

D: Okay, so now go back to your room and look up at your mother. [pause] And now what's happening?

I wanted to give her an opportunity to road test whatever change had occurred.

C: [pause] She's so sad.

D: Yes. And can you notice what happens to you when you allow her sadness to be hers?

C: I'm sad, but it's okay.

D: Yes. You can give her the freedom to be sad. And this is a freedom for you too, no?

C: Yes. [pause] It's okay.

D: Okay, well, you can return to this room now, bringing with you the sensation of having had a restful nap.

Five weeks later, when the couple returned for their last appointment, Carrie told me she no longer heard the voice and no longer felt "the oppressive weight" she'd always carried around. She felt more confident, more sure of what to do, and her worry was, she said, "within normal limits."

## Introduce New Ideas and Possibilities via Distinctions

Can you tell the difference between quitting and acceptance? This is the question I posed to Mac's family when they accused him of throwing in the towel in his fight against cancer (see Chapter 2). The difference depended, the family and I decided, on how long he ended up living. If he still had two good years in him, then he was clearly a quitter. But if death was imminent, then the attitude they'd been interpreting as "giving up" would actually be one of "letting go," of acceptance. Since no one could predict with any certainty the amount time he had left, they couldn't tell for sure whether they were seeing a sign of weakness or of strength.

Had I gone head to head with Mac's family, trying to force them to see Mac in a more positive light, I'm sure I'd have failed, for they would have had to defend their view from my efforts to change it. But when I asked whether they were able to distinguish their perspective from one that was just a thin dividing line away from it, they were initially stumped. All of us got curious *together,* looking closely at the belief they'd been holding *in relation to* one they'd previously not considered. What better way to safely explore an alternative understanding, to comfortably entertain a new possibility?

With Mac's family, the teasing apart took place in the realm of ideas—we had an intellectual discussion that helped clarify the time-based difference between quitting and acceptance. But often, clients can only discover answers through some kind of in-the-world *experience.*[17]

Kaisha, a therapist on one of my practicum teams, was seeing a couple in their mid-twenties—Marty and Glynis—who were fighting over Marty's use of prescription and nonprescription drugs. Two years earlier, a psychiatrist had started him on antipsychotic medication to control hallucinations and paranoia. He'd responded relatively well, but he often made his own dosage decisions, and he'd continued his recreational use of marijuana and LSD. Glynis, frightened that he was putting himself at risk for another psychotic break, tirelessly urged him to follow the doctor's recommended dosages and to stop using illegal substances. Marty just as tirelessly reminded her that she'd known how much he loved getting high when she met him, so why did she think he would change now? He'd recently stopped dealing drugs and was attending a community college, but this wasn't enough for her.

Kaisha empathized with Glynis's fear, as well as with Marty's frustration at having his life so closely dictated by his doctor's orders and his wife's admonitions. She then asked Marty whether he could tell if his passion for taking illegal drugs was a commitment to getting high or a commitment to achieving the independence of adulthood. He said he wasn't sure, so we suggested that the couple conduct an experiment to find out. As long as Glynis continued to try to save Marty from his drugs, he could never know what was inspiring his pull toward them. But if she left him to his own devices, they would have an opportunity to discover whether he truly was devoted to getting high or was actually devoted to having the freedom to make up his own mind about what was best for his future.

Marty agreed straightaway to the experiment, but Glynis, living in daily fear that Marty's next trip would take him back over the edge into psychosis, was more cautious. Exhausted by continually trying to protect Marty from himself, she needed the break the experiment would provide, but she wasn't sure she was quite ready to find out that the man she'd married wasn't capable of growing up and being a father to the children she wanted to bear. If Marty discovered he was simply a devoted druggie, she'd be forced to make a decision she'd been avoiding. Despite such risks, Glynis decided to give the experiment a shot, and over the next several weeks, they were surprised to learn that what Marty had thought was simply an insatiable desire for drug-induced reverie was actually a strong desire to make decisions he knew for sure were *his*.

The distinction we offered the couple contrasted their current understanding of their dilemma with an idea that hadn't previously been floated as a possibility. As a consultant on another case, I suggested that the therapist similarly juxtapose a new notion with an established belief and then invite his client to discover which one better fit her experience. I thought of the distinction as a win-win safety net for someone who was pinning all her hopes on a single solution.

Ted, a Christian counselor, had been working for a while with Fay, a deeply religious woman, but they hadn't made much progress. Feeling ever more desperate, Fay had concluded that she must be possessed by evil spirits, and she'd asked Ted to find her an exorcist. Although his denomination didn't recognize the legitimacy of possession and exorcism, Ted in fact knew an exorcist he considered reputable and sincere, someone who wouldn't exploit Fay and wouldn't charge for his services. Nevertheless, he was reluctant to send her to see him.

Swirling in tragedy and despair, Fay was desperate for some relief. But what would happen if she were to pin her last shreds of hope on the exorcism and it then made no difference? Ted didn't want to set her up to experience still more tragedy, but neither did he want to leave her feeling despondent, without any options, or to put her at risk of finding, on her own, an exorcist who was sleazy or disrespectful. Was there a way, he wondered, to get her out of what appeared to be a lose-lose situation?

I thought Ted had a good shot at setting up a win-win scenario if, before he told Fay about the exorcist, he reminded her of Job's trials. Satan put Job through hell, but he had permission from God to do so. God was behind the scenes the whole time, testing Job's faith. Did Fay know for sure the source of her problems? She'd assumed— for good reason, given the extent of her pain and loss—that she was possessed by evil spirits, but it was also possible that her tragedies were a spiritual test. Like Job, she could be suffering at the hands of God.

Of course, she probably couldn't, by herself, differentiate the cause of her suffering, which is why her idea of the exorcism was so timely and perfect. What better way of discovering the source of her misery? If, once she'd been exorcized, she felt liberated and strong, able once again to feel the power of God's love, she'd know she'd been cleansed of demonic powers. If, however, she still felt miserable, she'd know she was, in fact, possessed by God. After all, an exorcism will only remove evil spirits, never the presence of the Divine. If she was being tested by God, she would know that her despair was a sign that God was keeping his eye on her and that she, like Job, must be one of His most loyal subjects.

With the safety net in place, Ted accompanied Fay to the exorcism, an event he later described as both dramatic and respectful. Fay felt she benefitted significantly from the ritual; soon after, she moved back to her home town, only slightly bothered, she later told Ted, by a couple of mischievous sprites.

### Practice Tai Chi Therapy

If you decide at some point to study tai chi chuan, the Chinese soft-style martial art, you'll learn not to waste your strength and time directly blocking your opponents' strikes. Instead, you'll develop the ability to move with the force of the blow, getting out of its way and steering it in a new direction.

But even if you never bother with the physical side of tai chi, you can adopt its principles when responding to your clients' problems. Rather than trying to directly block or stop a symptom, you can find a way to flow with it, inviting it to move in a new direction.

A former student, Cary, called me about a client, Krystal, who had recently gone through detox and completed a twenty-eight-day addictions treatment program. Currently finishing up her outpatient sessions with Cary, Krystal was doing a great job staying clean, and she was back on her feet, but she was getting stressed out by a sexual issue—something she hadn't mentioned in any of the daily inpatient group-therapy sessions or during their previous outpatient appointments.

Krystal had divulged to Cary that for the six months prior to hitting bottom, she'd resorted to hooking as a means of supporting her habit. Now, whenever she and her boyfriend started to have sex, she'd be okay for the first five minutes, but after that she'd get creeped out. His hands would begin feeling like the hands of the Johns and, if she didn't stop and turn on the lights, she'd start smelling and tasting the Johns, too.

I suggested to Cary that he talk to Krystal about what happens when you hit bottom, about being able to reassess your life and make choices about how to be different. But to get to a new place with yourself, you need help. The people in treatment programs provide helping hands from above, reaching out to grasp your hand, so you can pull yourself up and out of your predicament. But there are also helping hands from below—the hands that remind you where you've been and encourage you to realize that you don't want to return there. Both sorts of hands are necessary. You might not know where to climb without the help from above, but you might forget how bad it was without the help from below, without the hands from below that help push you up and out of the pit. A time may come when you don't need to feel the hands from below anymore, but right now they are helping you not return to using, and so it can be so good to feel those helping hands gently support you in your new life, preventing you from falling back.

Cary told me later that when he passed on these ideas to Krystal, her face brightened and glowed like he hadn't seen before. She told him she didn't think she needed another appointment, and when he called to follow up, she said things were "now going fine."

By suggesting to Krystal that the sensation of the Johns' hands could actually *help* her with her continuing recovery, Cary was redirecting, rather than attempting to block, her symptom. I made a similar tai chi move with someone I mentioned earlier in the chapter— a woman who wanted to stop, as she put it, obsessing about a former boyfriend. Whenever she was alone or was bored at work, she'd find herself daydreaming about him, wishing she could be with him, despite his being involved with someone new, despite knowing rationally that he'd make a horrible husband. Rather than encouraging her to try to block or stop her thoughts, I suggested that she jump into her fantasies with both feet and, once inside them, expect to discover something unexpected. She might, I offered, imagine herself gazing into his eyes longingly, looking deeply and searchingly until she saw herself reflected in his pupils. If she looked still deeper, looking more and more closely at her reflection, she could move all the way into *her* thoughts, into *her* experience, discovering something about herself that had previously escaped her notice.

## Attend to Differences

I spoke earlier about refusing to offer "How-was-your-week?" therapy. Let me say more about what I meant. If you begin your sessions with this or an analogous question, then, unless your clients are just about ready to stop coming to see you, you risk getting a detailed accounting of the last seven days of irritations and inequities. If your clients consider it essential to fill you in on every detail of what's been happening, and if you think it's essential to honor their assumption, then you and they will likely be pleased with their having the opportunity to tell the latest plot twists of their ongoing story. But if the ongoingness of the story is about how things have remained pretty much the same, then nothing in your session will lend itself to altering their relationship with their problem, and nothing will head them in the direction of not needing to come back to see you. So you (and they) shouldn't be surprised if the conversation you have this time isn't demonstrably different from the one you had last or the one you'll have next. Or next. Or next. Or next.

I often need an initial session, maybe two, to get a good insider's sense of what's going on with my clients and to etch out a therapeutic direction. But once my clients and I have an idea where we're headed and I've begun offering intraventions—reframes, hypnotic experiences of various kinds, suggestions for some kind of between-session data-gathering or experimenting—then my curiosity about their week extends only to the ways in which it has or hasn't been *different*. Are my clients noticing change in their situation? If they aren't, I listen carefully to their descriptions of what's been happening, ready to pick up on something that hasn't made it onto their radar.

Too many times, I've watched a therapist ask clients about any differences they've noticed since their previous appointment and, when they come up dry, take them at their word and stop listening for indications of change. I'm not suggesting you pester your clients, but just because they haven't noticed anything new doesn't mean you should assume nothing's cooking. In some ways, you're in a better position than they are to discover important differences—not because you're "a professional," but because of the perspective you gain by being absent from their lives for a week or more at a time.

I must have been thirteen or fourteen, old enough to be smarter than I thought I was. Home by myself, recovering from the stomach flu, I hadn't felt quite good enough to make it to school that day. But by mid-morning my appetite had returned, and I started looking for something to eat. A rectangular pan on the counter caught my eye, and there, inside, I discovered a little over half of one of my mother's tantalizing homemade cakes. What better way to further my recovery than to indulge a little?

My mother, I knew, wouldn't approve. Heading out the door that morning, she'd recommended dry toast and room-temperature ginger ale. Blahh! My brothers and dad had already dug in while I'd been sick, so I felt entitled to a sizable portion, but I knew that if I cut myself a square piece, the current straight edge of the remaining cake would be compromised, and Mom would come home and discover what I'd done. Wanting to stay out of trouble, I looked for a way of creating a win-win situation—a none-the-wiser mother and a cake-the-fuller son.

Taking a knife, I cut all the way across the width of the rectangular pan, shaving off a three-quarter-inch line of cake. Folded up, the result was the equivalent of a nice moderate square, and, best of all, it came out of the pan consequence-free. Comparing the new edge of the remaining cake with the original one, I knew I was safe. No way Mom would recognize such a small shift in position.

An hour or two later, I returned to the kitchen and, feeling hungry and smug, I made my first of three mistakes. After liberating another three-quarter-inch line of cake, I assessed the likely undetectability of my pilfering by comparing the straight edge I'd just created with the one that had resulted from my most recent cut, rather than with the original edge. Can you tell that history wasn't my best subject? Or math? I failed to recognize that I'd created a *progression* of changes.

Twice more returning for further sweet sustenance (three-quarters of an inch at a time), I repeated the same comparison error. Monitoring only successive, rather than cumulative, differences, I reassured myself that my thin-sliced enjoyments would remain my little secret. Imagine my guilty surprise just before dinner, then, when I heard an edgy rising tone in my mother's voice as she called my name from the kitchen: "*Douglas?!*" Busted!

If your clients make a series of small changes but don't keep track of their cumulative effect, the overall difference may fall below their perceptual threshold. That's where you come in. Anytime my clients describe an action, thought, or feeling I haven't heard before, I ask them to compare their recent experience with what it likely would have been prior to their beginning therapy: "If you'd encountered the same circumstances two or three months ago, do you think you'd have responded the same way?" My change-based curiosity organizes my listening, so I'm always ready to hear something I haven't before. But I never try to convince my clients that they are in some way changing. If we determine that no differences are apparent (yet), I search around for a way of making sense of that and proceed accordingly. However, if they agree that something novel has indeed happened, we can then establish this new state of affairs as a jumping-off point for the *next* change: "Now that you've found a new way of doing *this,* what's next?"

### Stir Time and Doubt into
### Negative Truth Claims

A therapist on one of my practicum teams, Ofri, started seeing the Strickers family shortly after the seventeen-year-old son, Brady, had begun making some remarkable changes—changes that continued and developed over the course of the therapy. For the first time, Brady was holding down and working hard at a job he liked, going to night school to prepare for taking his GED, avoiding the friends with whom he'd gotten arrested, and helping his younger brother with some school-related problems. Nevertheless, his mother was worried he might slip back into his old ways. "My son has sticky fingers," she said vehemently in the fourth or fifth session. "He's a thief, and nothing we've tried has made a damn bit of difference."

If Ofri had accepted this statement, either by asking questions about it (e.g., "How long have you known this?" or "What sorts of things haven't worked?") or by changing the subject (e.g., "What *have* you been successful in making different?"), she'd have also been accepting the assumption that nothing Brady had been accomplishing in the previous couple of months had affected his proclivity for stealing. Instead, she and I found a way for her to wonder with the family whether Brady's various changes might have already begun (or might soon begin) to influence the stickiness of his fingers.

In describing Brady as a thief, his mom was making a truth claim about him—a description that supersedes time and context. I'm quite willing to accept positive truth claims about my clients (whether opined by the clients themselves or by someone else), as long as they support the idea that the clients are capable of changing. Had Brady's mom, for example, talked about how tenderhearted or smart her son had always been, Ofri could have tied these qualities into his ability to continue making important changes. But negative truth claims get in the way of therapeutic transformations.

- "I'm just a depressed person—it's who I am."
- "We never get along."
- "He's got one hell of a temper."
- "I never know what to do when she gets like this."

If accepted at face value, such statements have the potential to wipe out the significance of any changes the clients have been experiencing. To help prevent this eventuality, I ask various questions designed to stir time and doubt into the conversation.[18]

- "What shifts, if any, have you noticed in your depression in the last couple of weeks? Any thoughts you haven't had before? Have you found yourself doing anything different when you're feeling down?"
- "Think back over how you've not been getting along the last little while. What's been different about your disagreements or fights? Are you arguing more or less? Louder or softer? Has the content shifted in some way? Any differences in how you feel while you're yelling?"
- "Have you caught any differences in his temper in the past month or so? A shorter fuse? Longer? More angry than usual? Less? Any new things he does or says just before or just after he's lost it?"
- "Okay, so she's gotten like this, what, two or three times in last several weeks? And you haven't known what to do, right? Have you noticed, recently, anything different in what you're thinking or feeling as you stand there, not knowing what to do?"

In each case, I don't directly challenge the content of what the clients say; rather, I look for possible variations or shifts within the overarching "truth" they present. Notice in the examples that I don't go in search of how things have *improved* since the beginning of therapy, only how they might have *changed*. If my clients were to think I was trying to steal away their truth claims, they'd naturally have to defend them from me. I protect them from having to do that by asking about variations, good *and* bad. I'm not concerned if they tell me their situation has gotten worse—the major challenge is to get it *moving*. I simply want to enliven the assumption that change in one part of their life makes it possible in others.

## Practice Respect

Before coming to see me, Angela and Jose had been to a string of professional helpers, looking for someone who could stop their eleven-year-old son, Bo, from vomiting. Three gastroenterologists, a couple of nutritionists, an acupuncturist, a few holistic medicine people, and a previous hypnotherapist had all failed to make a difference. I commented on how difficult it must have been for the parents to reach out for help one more time, given how discouraging their journey to date had been. Both of them teared up.

The problem had started eight months earlier, they told me, when Bo contracted a bad case of stomach flu. After a week or ten days, he recovered from the virus, but his stomach had never returned to normal. He threw up almost daily, sometimes as often as six or eight times, and even when he was able to keep down his food, he often felt nauseated. An honor student and an accomplished hockey player, Bo had missed a lot of school and team practices.

Near the beginning of the first session, I told the family about a guy I knew growing up who was able to vomit on cue. His skill proved invaluable when, for example, he and his friends wanted to get into a fair or concert without having to pay. In front of the ticket booth, just before the attendant took his money, he'd double over and start losing his most recent meal. In the ensuing chaos, he and his buddies would jump the turnstile and make a run for it, disappearing into the crowd.

I suggested to Bo that his ability to throw up was an essential part of staying healthy. Even if he never made use of it to create a distraction at a county fair, it would no doubt come in handy in other ways. If he were to eat spoiled food, for example, he'd need to be able to unswallow it, and if someone were to jump him and demand his money, wouldn't it be nice, instead of giving the guy his wallet, to offer him the lunch he'd been digesting for the last couple of hours? The rest of the time—when vomiting *wasn't* necessary for ensuring his well-being—his body might as well discover a way for the nausea to turn into some other kind of feeling, a feeling that wouldn't trigger his gag reflex.

I also made a point of contradicting the professionals who'd told Bo (and his parents) that his problem was all in his head. "If that were the case," I said, "your stomach wouldn't feel so crummy, right? If the lousy feeling is down there under your sternum, why don't we go ahead and listen to what your body's saying? Who knows how the feeling will change once we invite it to? Certainly all the professionals you've seen wouldn't have a clue. I don't know either, and neither, probably, do you. But your stomach can discover just how it will shift and then let us in on whatever it figures out."

We did a couple of sessions of hypnosis, during which I invited the feeling at the top of his stomach to start changing in some way, perhaps by becoming more concentrated, perhaps by shifting position or quality, perhaps by getting bigger and bigger. I told him about picking up a deflated balloon once that looked almost black. As I blew it up, the color got lighter and lighter, to where in the end it was almost lavender. Had he done any science experiments in school, taking some dark dye and adding a drop or two to a gallon of water? Amazing what happens to a color when the molecules that make it up are spread far, far apart.

Bo and I discovered that his nausea changed when the feeling started increasing in volume. The quality of it, he said, remained the same, but as it expanded, it got distributed so widely that he could no longer find it in any one place in his body. I joked about it expanding so far that the moon would soon be getting the urge to barf.

Within a few weeks, the vomiting all but stopped, and Bo returned full-time to school and to playing hockey. Several months later, Angela called, upset. Bo had, the evening before, confessed that back when he was recovering from the flu, he'd been scared by how far he'd fallen behind in school, and he hadn't felt strong enough to get back on the hockey team. To cope, he'd faked out her and Jose, sticking his fingers down his throat when they were elsewhere in the house and lying about vomiting when they weren't around to see or hear. He'd wanted to buy himself a little adjustment time, but his hoax got out of hand, and once they'd started traipsing around to all the professionals, he hadn't known how to stop it.

Angela and Jose handled the revelation with poise and acceptance, but they were troubled by the news. I pointed out that Bo, in choosing to divulge his secret to them, was making sure he continued to handle difficulties without resorting to either real or fake vomiting. They were relieved to realize he'd taken an important step forward.

Obviously, the hypnosis wasn't responsible for bringing an end to Bo's stomach problems, given that he had started feeling better several months before coming to see me. But what about his ruse? How did he decide it was time to drop it? Perhaps he was just finally ready to move on, but I suspect that Bo's change—his letting go of faking everybody out—had something to do with having his feeling respected. I defended him against the charge that he had something wrong with his head, I empathized with his parents' exhaustion and fear, and, in no rush to get rid of the "nausea" and "throwing up," I showed my appreciation for how his body worked. Such respect can help clients change without losing face.

## Help Your Clients Save Face

Imagine having spent several hundred thousand dollars at various medical centers, trying to find the cause for the excruciating pain in your pelvic area. After countless tests and procedures, you're told that the pain is all in your head, and you're advised to go see a shrink. Here, finally, is the official confirmation of what your spouse has suspected all along—you really are crazy, after all. No wonder you allowed your faux medical problems to wipe out the savings and retirement accounts, max out all the credit cards, and create such a long line of bill collectors! Your parents and siblings agree with your spouse's assessment, dismissing you as a flake. And the pain, which continues unabated, is unpredictable and unforgiving. Despite your desire to get back into the work force, it holds you back and keeps you down, leaving you helpless and hopeless.

And then you happen upon me. In what kind of position are you going to be if our hypnotherapy sessions start making a difference? What's your spouse and family going to think if, after getting to the brink of financial ruin, you're able to start feeling better after a few sessions? Won't this just be further proof you're a nutcase? A lessening of the pain will only increase their (and your own) recriminations. After all, if the pain can change this dramatically this quickly, why the hell didn't you go this route *before* digging yourself a financial and emotional grave?

If your sessions with me *fail* to make much of a difference, you'll have to contend with renewed despair and hopelessness, but at least your integrity will remain somewhat intact. The intractability and intensity of your pain indicate that it is both real and outside your control. My failure to help may thus allow it (and you) to get a kind of grudging nod of legitimacy from your spouse and family, a recognition that you aren't *choosing* to be miserable.

Any therapeutic choices I make must take such considerations into account. If I can't help you save face, how can you be freed up to change?[19] I thus must begin by legitimizing you and your experience. As I did with Bo, I'll tell you that, if the pain were in your head, you'd be having *head*aches—since it is burning and piercing there in your pelvic area, then, obviously, that's where it must be.

The next step will be to legitimize the possibility of change. I'll want you to appreciate that the pain can be real *and* still be capable of transforming. To put flesh on this idea, I'll tell you stories of other clients of mine who've had weird pain-shifting experiences, and I'll suggest the possibility that you, too, will experience something similar. I'll explain that the pain might move to a different location, intensify for a while, or become more concentrated or more dissipated. Or its quality may change somehow, becoming more aching than burning or more pulsing than piercing, or developing inner variations in the sensation, with the middle, say, feeling different than the edges. And so on.

The final step will be to protect any changes in the pain by legitimizing *mystery*. I'll make note of all the unanswered questions surrounding your pain, detailing all that still remains unknown, and then I'll ask you whether it would be okay, at least for a while, for your body to continue keeping you in the dark about whatever changes begin to happen. Can you tolerate the mystery? Can you put up with the possibility of your pain beginning to change and your not even initially being aware of it? If you can, I'll then ask if you'd be willing, once you *do* begin to notice the changes, to keep them to yourself, at least for the time being. Would it be okay to begin feeling better without letting your spouse and family know?

In short, I'll do everything I can to ensure that changes in your pain don't undermine your integrity. I'll want to help you save face with your spouse and your family, but also with yourself. Only then, I figure, will you be able to feel some degree of safety about venturing forward.

## Help Your Clients Lose Track of Their Problem

Kevin's problem had already gotten a little better before his first appointment with me—a change he attributed to the medication his doctor had prescribed. Up until a few months earlier, he'd been unable, for about a year, to drive anywhere with anyone (including just himself) without extreme discomfort. Now, taking the medication, he was okay driving alone or with his wife, but anytime he got in the car with anyone else, he'd become overwhelmingly fearful of having an attack of diarrhea. As he drove or was driven, he'd continually scout for public restrooms, just in case he needed to stop.

On those occasions when he knew in advance that he'd be driving with someone other than (or in addition to) his wife, he'd start feeling panicky as soon as the plans had been made. He had, during a few different trips to a restaurant or concert, found it necessary to stop along the way and run to a bathroom. Having made it to the toilet, he'd usually discover he didn't have to go, after all, but this didn't keep him from needing to stop again a few miles further down the road, and it didn't keep him from feeling edgy, sweaty, and embarrassed.

A friend had referred him to me after a gastroenterologist found nothing wrong. We met for a total of six sessions over three and a half months, the middle four of which involved hypnosis. During our sessions, I helped him differentiate the "I've-gotta-poop" feeling in his lower intestines from the "I'm-worried-I've-gotta-poop" feeling in his stomach. His body knew how to digest food, I said, but it also knew how to digest the feeling of worry, as well as any rogue thought (such as, "It's too far to the next bathroom"). Just as his digestive system could break a chunk of food into its component molecules, absorbing what was necessary to fuel his metabolism, so, too, could he digest a thought or feeling or experience, allowing it to be automatically teased apart into component parts and used to fuel his sense of humor, his compassion, his curiosity about others in the car, his sense of peace with himself. Any indigestible bits would, of course, serve as fiber, chauffeuring the digestible components through his system.

Kevin responded well to our sessions. As his relationship to his fear changed, so did the fear itself. By the time of our last session, held almost two months after the previous one, he'd had many opportunities to be in cars with other people. Unlike before, he hadn't avoided taking any trips, and he no longer found it necessary to make pit stops. He felt like he'd experienced "a lot of success," but he was still often thinking about the *possibility* of having a problem, and he wondered if he would always have such thoughts, if he'd ever be free of them. Was there anything he could do, he asked, to safeguard against the problem returning? Were the suggestions liable to wear off at some point?

Great questions, eh? Like other clients who've achieved significant relief and, as a result, feel a little shaky about whether their good fortune will endure, Kevin could easily have started an egg-shell vigilance in an effort to protect the gains he'd made. To help ensure that this wouldn't be necessary, I did what I could to help him relax into trusting his body's ability to know what to do, even if he himself (that is, his *i*) didn't have a clue what that entailed. We live in a free country, I said, where free speech is protected by law. Surely your mind and body deserve the same respect, the same rights. Rather than trying to protect yourself by striving to stifle, subdue, or banish an unsettling thought or an uncomfortable feeling, why not let it come along for the ride? Give it the freedom to express itself, knowing that such freedom will then allow it to transform, to be digested, to go on its way.

"I could imagine," I said to Kevin, "that a hypnotic suggestion might somehow 'wear off' if it didn't fit with you, if it felt like it had been imposed on you." Mixing metaphors, I went on: "This is no different from what your digestive system does with indigestible fiber—it refuses to absorb it." But I reassured him that the stuff I had said to him during the hypnosis was as much his as mine, so I saw no reason why, at this point, it would get excreted. If it did, we'd just need to find a different way for his body to carry on its newly acquired digestive habits, but I didn't anticipate this happening. I then switched metaphors again:

> I think of therapeutic change like rearranging furniture. If you discover that your couch works better over there than over here, and then you reposition the chairs and the lights and the tables, if your living room has better flow after you've done all that, then the space somehow "fits" you better. When it fits like that, you don't then go to bed at night, concerned you'll wake up the next morning and everything will have shifted back the way it was. Why would it? Same deal with hypnosis. If a new arrangement of ideas or responses works better for you, it feels more in keeping with who you are, right? It gives you better flow. So no need to bother wondering if it's going to move back to the old way when you aren't looking. If you end up wanting to make another shift in the future, sure, why not? But your body now knows how to deal with those feelings in your stomach, so if you started feeling the butterflies fluttering again, your body knows how to go into digestion mode.

I never want to leave my clients with the impression, or even the hope, that they won't at some point encounter again whatever brought them to see me in the first place. They may not, but to hold out the impossible possibility of a "pure" separation from their problem—that is, that our work together will result in a "cure"—would only heighten the problem's significance and increase the probability of its continuing to be an issue. Instead, I offer the prospect of a *connected* separation—a relationship with the problem that gives it the freedom to transform *and* the liberty to visit again in the future. That way, if it drifts away and never returns, they'll be pleasantly surprised, and if it comes back, they'll be well prepared to once again expedite its unraveling. In the meantime, as the problem shifts in quality and intensity, moving from foreground prominence to background irrelevance, my clients are given the opportunity to venture beyond the symptom-defining boundaries within which they've been living. This is the shape, the relational freedom, of therapeutic change.

# Glossary

**association**  A process of connection. See *connection* and *dissociation*.

**categorization**  A result of the associational nature of cognition. When you distinguish something in perception and/or language, you determine what it *isn't* by separating it from its surroundings, by defining it as a distinct object. Simultaneously, you establish what it *is* by categorizing it—connecting it with other things with which it shares something in common. Such associational bundles can themselves be distinguished and named as consciously discernible objects. But we also make connections without recognizing that we're doing it. These unnamed or tacit categories still affect how we make sense of (attach meaning to) things, but we aren't aware that it is happening. See *context suggestion*.

**concordance**  (< Latin *con*, together + *cord-*, heart: *concorda-re*, to be of one mind.) A heart-and-mind connection (a) between two (or more) people (say, a therapist and a client); (b) between a person and him- or herself; and/or (c) between a person and his or her problem.

(a) When a therapist and a client are in concordance, the client finds it unnecessary to keep track of or to protect the boundary between them. Such rapport or trust facilitates the client's concording with him- or herself and/or his or her problem.

(b) When a client is in concordance with him- or herself, the *i* stops distinguishing itself as separate from the rest of the self, so the usual mind/body split of conscious awareness doesn't bother getting marked as relevant.

(c) When a client is in concordance with his or her problem, the problem isn't distinguished as Other, as something to be eradicated. This creates the necessary conditions for therapeutic change.

**connection**   Given the associational nature of mind, all purposeful cognitive acts create connections. The more connected you are to someone or something, the less you notice or care about the differences—the boundary—between you and him or her or it.

**connected separation**   A nonpurposeful separation that develops within the context of a connection. If you're holding onto something and won't or can't let go, I'd be crazy to try to grab it away from you, as that would only heighten its significance for you. When you trust that I won't do that, you don't have to be as vigilant in holding onto it, and if, then, you become captivated by (connected to) something *else,* your relationship with the original something can become a connected separation. If that happens, you'll lose track of it, let go of it, forget about it, stop caring about it, or not be bothered with it. Such connected separations create *gaps of insignificance.*

**context suggestion**   A suggestion that offers a context-setting idea outside the purview of conscious awareness. If I offer you a choice between two or three possibilities and you pick one of them, your choice will be delimited—contextualized—by the range of the presented options. If I tell you three stories back to back, the juxtaposition makes it possible for your understanding to be similarly contextualized by the not-consciously-noticed connection between them.

**dissociation**   A process of separation. Dissociation creates divisive relationships between the objects it differentiates. Conscious awareness is entirely dependent on dissociation—you couldn't distinguish objects in perception and language without separating them from what they aren't. In addition, consciousness—your dissociated sense of "self"—is a reflexive artifact of this process. See *i.*

**distinction**   A relationship established by separating *this* from *that* or *this* from *not-this.* A distinction connects what it separates.

**gap of insignificance**   The only separation within the associative web of mind that doesn't create an out-of-awareness connection.

**hypnosis**   An intrapersonal relationship in which the *i* stops bothering to demarcate itself as separate from (and in control of) the rest of the self, altering the experience of the usual *i*-constructed boundaries between mind and body. See *concordance.*

**hypnotherapy**   A way of inviting and using intrapersonal concordance to introduce freedom into the client-problem relationship.

*i*   The homunculus up there in your head that, in pure Cartesian fashion, identifies itself as the locus of selfhood—as the director, dictator, and brains of the operation. This is the self-within-the-Self—the "i" within the I—that you distinguish when you say or think, "I am having trouble controlling my thoughts," "I am feeling better," "I am no longer concerned about my knee," or "I don't like myself."

**intravention**   (< Latin *intra,* on the inside, within + *venire,* to come: to come from within.) Suggestions for change that arise from and fit within each client's idiosyncratic circumstances. Designed to transform, rather than stop or eradicate, client problems, intraventions start occurring to you and making sense when you're able to use your metaphoric imagination to cross the self-other boundary separating you from your clients.

**invitation**   Contrary to popular assumption, your job is not to *induce* your clients into a dissociative hypnotic state, but, rather, to *invite* them into an associative relationship (into concordance) with themselves.

**metaphoric imagination**   Treating or experiencing *this* as if it were *that*. Your metaphoric imagination kicks in at the movies (and while reading novels) when you find yourself responding to the storyline as if you were one (or more) of the characters. It kicks in during therapy when you're able to imagine yourself as your clients, making sense of their thoughts, feelings, choices, and sensations from inside their experience. Such metaphoric understanding is necessary if you are to offer more than knee-jerk empathic comments and questions.

**of one mind**   A relationship of concordance in which the usual *i*-defined boundaries of the self lose significance.

**relational freedom**   Not freedom *from* but freedom *within* the context of a relationship.

**separated connection**   An inadvertent disjunctive relationship (between two or more people, or between a person and some aspect of his or her experience) that results from a purposeful attempt to negate or otherwise separate from someone or something feared or hated.

**separation**   A division created in one of two ways:

(a) When a distinction is drawn or a boundary is imposed. Such separations simultaneously create connections. See *separated connection*.

(b) When a connection *there* makes possible a gap of insignificance *here*. See *connected separation*.

**therapeutic change**   A freeing transformation in the relationship between clients and their problem, such that the problem shifts in meaning, significance, duration, intensity, or quality.

**thingking**   Another name for conscious thought, which, slicing experience into isolable objects, treats things, rather than relationships, as if they were the primary building blocks of mind.

**trance**   (< Latin *trans*, across + *ire*, to go: the action or fact of passing across or through.) You go into trance when the usual boundary between your *i* and the rest of you is crossed, allowing your mind to become embodied and your body to become mindful. With your *i* not (for a time) being distinguished as the owner and ruler of your experience, your perceptions of yourself can shift significantly. See *concordance, hypnosis, i,* and *of one mind*.

**unanimity**   (< Latin *unus*, one + *animus*, mind.) When you and your clients are in concordance and they agree with what you're offering them, they find it possible to take what you're suggesting and run with it. Some hypnosis theorists, making use of their best thingking, take this relational phenomenon and treat it as an encapsulated trait—named "suggestibility"—that supposedly resides inside of individuals.

**unconscious**   Relationships remain unconscious—that is, out of awareness—until they are named or otherwise isolated and reified as discernable things. Given the associative web of mind, the processes and contexts of experience are necessarily relational, and, thus, unconscious.

# Notes

## Acknowledgments

1. Here's what I wrote: "This book recasts the theory and practice of hypnosis and therapy within a *relational* understanding of language, self, and mind."

## Introduction

1. To protect the anonymity of my clients, I've given them all pseudonyms and have changed identifying details about their lives.
2. I use this construction—clients (plural)/problem (singular)—throughout the book. Part of the reason is stylistic—it helps me keep my pronoun references clear ("they" consistently refers to the clients; "it," to their problem), without the his-and-her clumsiness that would result from making "clients" singular. But it also fits with my way of working. As you'll soon discover, I'm always thinking and acting relationally, whether eight people come to an appointment or one. Thus, even if I have only an individual in my office, I'm taking into consideration his or her relationships with others, wondering who else has a stake in his or her changing. He or she, then, with his or her problem, is often not the only client in the picture, even if I never actually meet the others who are important in his or her life. (See what I mean?)

## Chapter One

1. Parts of this chapter first appeared in an article I wrote for the January/February, 1999, issue of the *Family Therapy Networker.*

2. According to Cardeña (1994), dissociation has been described by personality theorists and clinical psychologists "in a least three distinct ways. First, dissociation is used to characterize semi-independent mental modules or systems that are not consciously accessible, and/or not integrated within the person's conscious memory, identity, or volition. Second, dissociation is viewed as representing an alteration in consciousness wherein the individual and some aspects of his or her self or environment become disconnected or disengaged from one another. And third, dissociation is described as a defense mechanism that effects [*sic*] such disparate phenomena as nonorganic amnesia, the warding off of current physical or emotional pain, and other alterations of consciousness, including chronic lack of personality integration, such as with Multiple Personality Disorder (MPD; referred to in the . . . DSM IV . . . as Dissociative Identity Disorder)" (p. 16).

3. Hilgard (1973) believed "daily life [to be] full of many small dissociations" (p. 406). I go further, viewing dissociation as the signature of consciousness. And, in contrast to Hilgard's position, I view *association,* not dissociation, to be the defining feature of hypnosis. As I explain below, hypnotic phenomena are *associated dissociations* or *connected separations.*

4. The following skit, written by Norman Stiles, aired August 24, 1998, on WPBT in Miami.

5. The following melodic line is from a piece called "Ontophony," composed by Michael O'Neill in 1995.

6. Said by Wallace Stevens.

7. By this I *don't* mean thinking that is full of metaphorical allusions. Rather, I am referring to metaphorically *shaped* thinking—associational thinking that separates things *in the service* of connecting them.

8. The distinction between "a part of" and "apart from" was highlighted by Kenneth Burke. More recently, Stephen Gilligan has used it in his discussions of hypnosis.

## Chapter Two

1. The therapists at the Mental Research Institute wrote about how difficulties in life turn into significant problems when people attempt to resolve them in ineffective ways. The problem, from their

perspective, is not the difficulty itself, but the clients' attempted solution. I am here going one step further, making the point that what
characterizes most such solution attempts is an effort to *negate* the
trouble.

2.  See Benjamin Hoff's (1983) *The Tao of Pooh* for a delightful explo-
    ration of this logic.

3.  This belief has also informed the style of this book. As you've no
    doubt noticed, I keep pulling the ideas out of (or folding them into)
    stories. I want you not only to critically examine what I'm saying,
    but also to absorb yourself in it.

4.  An earlier description of the following case was published as a chap-
    ter ("The Strength to Swallow Death") in the edited book, *Tales from
    Treating Families* (Thomas & Nelson, 1998).

5.  In Chapter 6, I explain the contextualizing effect of telling such
    stories.

6.  As I point out in Chapter 6, the juxtaposing of alternative possibil-
    ities creates an out-of-awareness connection between them—a tacit
    category that offers a contextualizing suggestion for change.

7.  I borrowed and adapted part of this "good-bye" story from Yapko
    (1990).

## *Chapter Three*

1.  For example, therapists can use diagnoses from the DSM-IV to sep-
    arate themselves from clients, to reassure themselves, in a "profes-
    sionally responsible" way, that they and their clients share nothing
    in common.

2.  In this instance, I was offering what I and my colleagues fondly call
    *dead* (as opposed to *live*) supervision. The therapist and I met once a
    week and talked about how his cases were proceeding.

3.  A slightly different version of this section first appeared in the
    March/April, 2001, issue of *Psychotherapy Networker.*

4.  Same translation for both: "What is that?"

5.  Bateson (2000) distinguished two patterns of dyadic relationship. In
    *symmetrical* interactions, the participants behave similarly—the
    more A does something, the more B responds in kind: The more you
    tell me about your life, the more I tell you about mine; the more you
    express sexual interest in me, the more I express sexual interest in

you; and so on. In *complementary* interactions, the participants' behaviors fit together, but they are *dis*similar—the more A does something, the more B responds in a different, but fitting, way: The more
you tell me about your life, the more I listen and ask questions; the
more you express sexual interest in me, the more I let you know that
I'm interested in your experience but not your affection; and so on.

6. And, sometimes, we may need not to be invested in getting our fee,
   either.

7. Some clients also believe this, but if you are effective in your work,
   you will help them change their minds. A couple came to our clinic
   looking for help with their sixteen-year-old daughter. At the beginning of their first appointment, they came back behind the one-way
   mirror to meet the team, and the husband asked us point blank:
   "How many of you are parents, and what are the ages of your kids?"
   When he learned that most of us had no children, he was disappointed, and he seriously considered leaving. He decided to stay,
   however, and, over the next two months, the situation with his
   daughter improved significantly. This is what he told us the night of
   his last appointment:

   > We needed other opinions. . . . I think what I asked when we first
   > came here was how many [of you] were *parents,* and . . . I thought
   > a lot [of you] *had* to be parents. But maybe [you] just had to [have]
   > insights into human behavior. So I guess it worked out well. We
   > just, we've asked a lot of questions and done a lot of things differ-
   > ently. . . . We thank you for your time. It has been good. It has
   > been good.

8. Probably no one is better at this than Meryl Streep. Take, for instance, how she "became" the real-life character of Roberta Guaspari
   for the movie *Music of the Heart.* The director of the film, Wes
   Craven, recalled how she prepared for her role: "The first time Meryl
   met Roberta at my office, . . . Meryl said to her, 'Let's go into
   wardrobe'. After ten minutes you could hear them laughing. And
   then they closed the door. They were in there for three hours, . . .
   and when [Meryl] came out, she had Roberta cold. It was like she
   had downloaded her" (Malanowski, 1999, p. 26).

9. As I mentioned in Chapter 1, the structure of metaphor embodies
   this paradoxical doubleness. A metaphor connects two things as

one—"love is a river"; "I am you"—but it can't assert the *unity* of the two things without simultaneously establishing their *separateness*. Metaphor can't cleave (together) without cleaving (apart). Metaphoric understanding, like metaphor, involves differentiation within fusion, separation within connection.

10. J. S. Bach wrote fifteen "two-part inventions" for harpsichord in 1722–1723.

11. Milton Erickson knew this better than anyone. See Haley (1973) for a variety of stories that depict Erickson's uncanny ability to grab hold of his clients' way of being.

12. The next week the class presented me with a new shirt. I've since found easier ways to build a wardrobe and safer ways to offer ideas.

13. As you probably remember from my interaction with the man wearing mirrored sunglasses, I also used empathy with him in a manipulative way: "So that puts you in a crummy place," I told him. "Not only do I have to tell you that I can't work with you, but the cops make me warn your wife that her life is in danger." Trying to protect myself from his possible wrath, I conveniently shifted the blame for my actions to the police. I was, at this point in the session, too unnerved to think and act therapeutically.

14. See Duncan, Hubble, and Miller (1997) for a captivating discussion about working with "impossible" cases.

15. Ericksonian utilization fits closely with this idea of intravention.

16. It was Bateson who first offered *frame* as a metaphor for context. Since the meaning of a piece of experience (an action, an idea, an emotion) depends on its context, reframing (recontextualizing) the experience transforms its meaning. See Chapter 1.

17. Kiri never directly mentioned being suspicious that rather than just masturbating, her husband was having an affair. I didn't broach the idea, figuring that I could do so later if it seemed relevant. It never did.

18. The Milan team called their reframes *positive connotations*. Later, they changed the term to *logical connotations*.

## Chapter Four

1. I dislike the physicality of the metaphor "resistance," and I also wish to avoid the connotations that accompany it. Clinicians have traditionally avoided taking responsibility for therapeutic failures

by pointing their fingers at their client's resistance. Milton Erickson, in contrast, approached hypnosis and therapy as opportunities to *utilize resistance.* See de Shazer (1984) for an excellent critique of the traditional position.

2. Alex Dominguez.

3. Gregory Bateson (1979, 2000) clearly detailed the problems of using quantitative metaphors to explain communicational phenomena.

4. If a teenage girl, say, tells you she doesn't want to work with you, you can always invite the parents to come in alone to talk about their concerns and to explore ways they can respond to her differently. Obviously, though, when court-ordered clients say they aren't interested in therapy, you can't call the judge and suggest that *he* or *she,* as the one concerned about the problem, be the one to attend sessions with you. Nevertheless, a friend of mine, William Rambo, who works with court-ordered sex offenders, never forces therapy on the men in his groups. Recognizing that he can do nothing unless they are oriented to getting something from him, he *invites* their participation (Rambo, 1999). The clients' probation officers require them to attend sessions, but Rambo doesn't push them to act in a predetermined way.

5. I misremembered some of the specifics. Erickson encouraged a twenty-year-old man with stunted growth and a stunted perspective of the world to hallucinate himself standing part way up a staircase. The man subsequently grew twelve, not six, inches. Erickson told David Cheek about the case, but he never submitted it to a journal, believing that "no respectable editor . . . would publish such an impossible thing" (Cheek, 1982, p. 282).

6. This is about as close as I'm comfortable getting to offering a suggestion that clients stop doing something—even a habit they've come in wanting to quit. I'm always sensitive to the possibility of further intensifying the separated connection between clients and their problem.

7. There are always exceptions. Milton Erickson once saw a couple who, because they wanted children, engaged (in their words) "in the marital union with full physiological concomitants each night and morning for procreative purposes" (Rossi, 1980, p. 448). Unfortunately, three years of committed effort had proved fruitless, so they came to Erickson for help. He told them he could help them but

that it would involve psychological "shock therapy." They agreed, so he said, "For three long years you have engaged in the marital union with full physiological concomitants for procreative purposes at least twice a day and sometimes as much as four times in twenty-four hours, and you have met with defeat of your philoprogenitive drive. *Now why in hell don't you fuck for fun and pray to the devil that she isn't knocked up for at least three months*" (Rossi, p. 449).

8. Yapko (1990, 1995) discusses common client misconceptions and offers excellent ideas for how to respond to them.

9. I suggest drawing on some of the ideas in this book, as well as from Kirsch (1990), Yapko (1995), T. X. Barber (1984), Erickson (1989), and O'Hanlon (O'Hanlon & Martin, 1992) in preparing your description.

10. A year and a half after I saw Keith, he told me that "ninety-nine-point-nine percent of the time, the thing you showed me [i.e., self-hypnosis] gets rid of my headaches [which used to last two days] in a minute or less."

11. See Chapter 6 for a detailed discussion of my therapeutic assumptions.

12. See Weakland, Fisch, Watzlawick, and Bodin (1974) for an excellent discussion of how solution attempts cause problems.

13. Even with such a change-focused approach, I'm still more patient than the brief-therapy intern my friend William Rambo once supervised. During their first pre-session, the young man aptly demonstrated his understanding of MRI therapeutic principles, noting that his first order of business with his clients was going to involve defining a clear problem on which to work. He left to see the case, having arranged to return for a post-session once the clients had gone home. Fifteen minutes later, he surprised William with a knock on his door. Asked if anything was wrong, he said no, the session was over. The clients had been unable to spout out a clear problem definition, so he told them he couldn't help them.

14. As I mentioned in my story about Jennifer, I don't offer after-hours on-call support, but I also don't refuse to talk to clients if they happen to reach me in my office when I have a few minutes to chat.

15. See Chapter 3, pp. 47–49.

16. The Milan Associates—Luigi Boscolo and Gianfranco Cecchin (Boscolo, Cecchin, Hoffman, & Penn, 1987)—were perhaps the first to articulate how problems can be viewed as solutions.

17. As I said at the beginning of the chapter, I don't find the notion of "motivation" helpful in making sense of how people go about taking action, but it was integral to Len's belief system, so I used it as a jumping-off point for exploring what he cared about and how he was changing.

18. Watzlawick (1982) made a cogent observation about what happens when clients involved in such therapy make no progress: "We all know the patient who after years of therapy has all the insight into his murky past he will probably ever have . . . and yet does not seem to benefit from having bathed in the crystal light of reason. Fortunately, a self-sealing explanation may be found for this phenomenon. It vindicates the true doctrine and is of great value to the therapist (and his bank account)—namely, that the lack of therapeutic results proves that the patient's past has not yet been sufficiently illuminated and that deeper therapy is still needed" (p. 149).

19. Some clinicians, such as Terr (1994) and Cheek (1994), have claimed that they can distinguish true from false memories; however, according to memory researchers such as Schacter (1996), "there is no research that allows clinicians or scientists to judge unequivocally the historical truth of a traumatic memory recovered in therapy" (p. 274).

## Chapter Five

1. In a conversation with Robert Rieber about the mind-body problem, Gregory Bateson illustrated his ideas with a Balinese painting of a man with a head at every joint—shoulders, elbows, wrists, knees, and ankles (Bateson & Rieber, 1989, p. 324). Bateson pointed out that the "Balinese don't have to think the way the occidentals think about bodies and minds" (p. 324). The man in the painting was "animated in every joint" (p. 323), each part of him "separately alive" (p. 324). As a hypnotherapist, I find it useful to think similarly about the mindfulness of people's bodies (e.g., Flemons & Shulimson, 1997).

2. Ernie Rossi does a nice job of creating no-fail hypnotic inductions.

3. My kids were both colicky as babies. Shelley and I took turns bouncing, dancing, and rocking Eric, always in search of the right speed, the right position to bring him some relief. When Jenna came

along, I tried something a little different. I realized that with Eric, the pace of our jostling was determined by us. What would happen, I wondered, if I adjusted my movements so that I was rhythmically in tune with *her?* Holding her in my arms, I moved in sync with her breathing—down as she wailed; up as she took a breath. I imagined her, as she cried, feeling "out of sorts," out of relationship, with herself and her surroundings—a significant change from her experience in the womb. My moving in time with her breathing would, I reasoned, help her feel less of the contrast between herself and her environment, which, in turn, might provide her a measure of comfort, a means for relaxing into a relationship with the arms cradling her and into a more relaxed relationship with herself. I had the sense that my method was helpful, but I haven't yet conducted a research study to empirically test my hunch. Nevertheless, I've continued to sync up with both kids' breathing whenever I want to help them relax or drift off to sleep. One afternoon when Jenna was three, she taught me that too much matching can create a mismatch. Laying next to her on her bed, trying to facilitate her taking a much needed, but not particularly wanted, nap, I started timing my exhales with hers. Before long, her breathing started to speed up. I thought this odd, but I followed suit, only to discover that she had been conducting her own little experiment. "Daddy," she suddenly said sternly, "don't copycat me!"

4. Even if talking takes my clients out of concordance with themselves, I will often still touch base with them every once in a while. You don't need to assume that your clients must stay absorbed 100% of the time. You can invite them into conversation, get the information you need, and then invite them back into hypnosis.

5. If a pathogenic double bind involves a situation where you're damned if you do and damned if you don't, a therapeutic double bind determines that you're blessed if you do and blessed if you don't.

6. Creating and offering therapeutic double binds requires you to think categorically. See Chapter 6, pp. 197–202.

7. Erickson often used hypnosis to help people vividly experience themselves at a point in the future when their problem was resolved or much improved. This technique was one of the inspirations for Steve de Shazer's nonhypnotic solution-focused therapy.

8. Sandra transcribed and analyzed the fourth session for her doctoral dissertation, a study that explores the links between hypnosis, Buddhist meditation, and oral poetry (Roscoe, 1996). In preparing this chapter, I relied heavily on her transcription, and I benefited from her insights.

## *Chapter Six*

1. Irving Kirsch has written a book (1990) and edited a volume (1999) on the vital role of expectancy in therapeutic transformations. If you are attending to your clients' *expectancy* about possibilities for change, you are similarly focusing on their *relationship* to their problem.

2. Bateson (1979) elucidated the cybernetic relationship between change and stability in living systems: "The rock's way of [surviving] is different from the way of living things. The rock, we may say, resists change; it stays put, unchanging. The living thing escapes change either by correcting change or changing itself to meet the change or by incorporating continual change into its own being. 'Stability' may be achieved either by rigidity or by continual repetition of some cycle of smaller changes, which cycle will return to a *status quo ante* after every disturbance. Nature avoids (temporarily) what looks like irreversible change by accepting ephemeral change" (p. 103). Following Bateson, Keeney (1983) made excellent use of this change/stability distinction in his mapping of family therapy. I prefer *continuity* over *stability,* as it better conveys, to my ear, the process, the ongoingness, of non-change.

3. As a means of creating distance, anger has its limitations. It works great as a short-term invitation to action, but if it persists too long, it becomes a kind of glue, a separated connection that binds the person to whatever he or she is angry at. By legitimizing anger (or any other emotional response), you help facilitate its changing.

4. Manny Perez-Campos and Sandra Roscoe.

5. I didn't, technically, misrepresent our actions. It *was* our last load; it's just that it was also our first.

6. Given the separative structure of consciousness, the *i* of necessity sets itself apart from the rest of the self and casts this rest-of-self as other. With people who self-mutilate or perpetrate some other kind of self-directed violence, this separation is simply more pronounced. Rather than just other, the rest-of-self becomes Other.

7. See Wilk (1985) and O'Hanlon and Wilk (1987) for a related discussion of this idea.

8. This is so universally recognized that a teenager or young adult who wants to be taken seriously will often start using, at this time, the more formal version of his or her name.

9. See pp. 181–183.

10. When I've talked about this case in professional settings, therapists have sometimes commented, I think correctly, on the similarities between this work and what a Gestalt therapist might do with the empty-chair technique. However, I didn't provide an empty chair (or in this case, an empty bed) and plop the father in it. I had no preconceived notion that Brent "needed" such an interaction with his dead father. I simply facilitated and then followed his creative lead. When the vibrations materialized into the figure of his father, I sought out various means for a therapeutic interaction, but I wasn't invested in Brent's discovering any particular shape.

11. After I got the idea to do this but before I broached it with Dierdre, I ran it by Shelley, my colleague and wife, to get a reality and gender check. She gave it a thumbs up.

12. Shelley Green and David Todtman.

13. Milton Erickson once said to Jay Haley, who was asking about the purposes of a client's symptom: "Your assumption is that it served other purposes. Have you ever thought about symptomatology wearing out in serving purposes and becoming an habitual pattern?" (Haley, 1985, p. 15).

14. And rightly so. Although the therapist was working from a strategic perspective, he wasn't heeding Jay Haley's (1976) counsel: "The therapist . . . will find it best if he does not deal explicitly with the issues in the marriage until he gets improvement in the child, the presenting problem. Rushing to the marriage as a problem can make therapy more difficult later" (p. 141).

15. I don't know whether Isadora's early-morning picture drawing helped free her from her nightmares. Thinking categorically when I made the suggestion, I was attempting to create the tacit idea that between the time she went to sleep and the time she woke up, her dreams would somehow be diminished by half. And if they could end up half the size, they could also become half as scary, right?

16. At a seminar in 1961, Milton Erickson (1986) told an assembled group of psychotherapists, "Your task is that of altering, not abolishing" (p. 104). See also the first epigraph of this chapter.

17. You may remember how, in Chapter 4, I described asking Rachel whether she could distinguish between solid and translucent fear.

18. I make sure, of course, to give clients the opportunity to answer the first question before I ask the second (see p. 75). O'Hanlon and Wilk (1987) also talk about introducing doubt (pp. 114–118).

19. Jay Haley (1985, p. 16) and Milton Erickson once had a conversation about helping clients move beyond their symptom:

    H: There is a nice phrase, "Often people need a graceful exit out of a symptom that no longer serves a purpose."

    E: In brief psychotherapy you always give them the graceful exit. In prolonged therapy you also do the same thing. You have to prolong therapy often because they fight so desperately against accepting a graceful exit.

# References

Barber, T. X. (1984). Changing "unchangeable" bodily processes by (hypnotic) suggestions: A new look at hypnosis, cognitions, imagining, and the mind-body problem. In A. A. Sheikh (Ed.), *Imagination and healing* (pp. 69–127). Farmingdale, NY: Baywood.

Bateson, G. (1979). *Mind and nature: A necessary unity.* Toronto: Bantam.

Bateson, G. (2000). *Steps to an ecology of mind.* Chicago: University of Chicago Press.

Bateson, G., & Rieber, R. W. (1989). Mind and body: A dialogue. In R. W. Rieber (Ed.), *The individual, communication, and society: Essays in memory of Gregory Bateson* (pp. 320–333). Cambridge: Cambridge University Press.

Bloom, P. B. (1994). Clinical guidelines in using hypnosis in uncovering memories of sexual abuse: A master class commentary. *International Journal of Clinical and Experimental Hypnosis, 42*(3), 173–178.

Boscolo, L., Cecchin, G., Hoffman, L., & Penn, P. (1987). *Milan systemic family therapy: Conversations in theory and practice.* New York: Basic.

Bowers, K. S. (1976). *Hypnosis for the seriously curious.* New York: W. W. Norton.

Cardeña, E. (1994). The domain of dissociation. In S. J. Lynn & J. W. Rhue (Eds.), *Dissociation: Clinical and theoretical perspectives* (pp. 15–31). New York: Guilford.

Cheek, D. (1982). Some of Erickson's contributions to medicine. In J. K. Zeig (Ed.), *Ericksonian approaches to hypnosis and psychotherapy* (pp. 281–286). New York: Brunner/Mazel.

Cheek, D. B. (1994). *Hypnosis: The application of ideomotor techniques.* Boston: Allyn and Bacon.

Combs, G., & Freedman, J. (1990). *Symbol, story, and ceremony: Using metaphor in individual and family therapy.* New York: W. W. Norton.

Coventry, M. (1996, Sept./Oct.). Quit pro quotes. *Utne Reader, 42*–44.

Crews, F. (1995). *The memory wars: Freud's legacy in dispute.* New York: New York Review of Books.

de Shazer, S. (1982). *Patterns of brief family therapy: An ecosystemic approach.* New York: Guilford.

de Shazer, S. (1984). The death of resistance. *Family Process, 23*(1), 11–17.

Duncan, B. L., Hubble, M. A., & Miller, S. D. (1997). *Psychotherapy with "impossible" cases.* New York: W. W. Norton.

Erickson, M. H. (1980). Further clinical techniques of hypnosis: Utilization techniques. In E. L. Rossi (Ed.), *The collected papers of Milton H. Erickson on hypnosis, vol. 1* (pp. 177–205). New York: Irvington.

Erickson, M. H. (1986). *Mind-body communication in hypnosis: The seminars, workshops, and lectures of Milton H. Erickson, vol. 3* (E. L. Rossi & M. O. Ryan, Eds.). New York: Irvington.

Erickson, M. H. (1989). Hypnosis. In S. R. Lankton (Ed.), *Ericksonian monographs, 5: Ericksonian hypnosis: Application, preparation, and research* (pp. 1–6). New York: Brunner/Mazel.

Erickson, M. H., & Rossi, E. (1980). Varieties of double bind. In E. L. Rossi (Ed.), *The collected papers of Milton H. Erickson on hypnosis, vol. 1* (pp. 412–429). New York: Irvington.

Fawcett, B. (1981). Tristram's book. *The Capilano Review, 19.*

Fisch, R., Weakland, J. H., & Segal, L. (1982). *The tactics of change.* San Francisco: Jossey-Bass.

Flemons, D. G. (1991). *Completing distinctions.* Boston: Shambhala.

Flemons, D. G., & Green, S. K. (1998). Hanging on to letting go: A relational approach to sex therapy. In W. J. Matthews & J. H. Edgette (Eds.), *Current thinking and research in brief therapy, vol. 2* (pp. 29–56). Philadelphia: Taylor & Francis.

Flemons, D. G., & Shulimson, J. (1997). Participating in the culture of cancer: A demilitarized approach to treatment. *Contemporary Hypnosis, 14*(3), 182–188.

Flemons, D. G., & Wright K. (1999). Many lives, many traumas: The hypnotic construction of memory. In W. J. Matthews & J. H. Edgette (Eds.), *Current thinking and research in brief therapy, vol. 3* (pp. 179–195). Philadelphia: Taylor & Francis.

Gilligan, S. (1987). *Therapeutic trances.* New York: Brunner/Mazel.

Green, S. (1994). The triplet who couldn't be: A matter of language. *Journal of Systemic Therapies, 13*(1), 51–64.

Haley, J. (1973). *Uncommon therapy: The psychiatric techniques of Milton H. Erickson, M.D.* New York: W. W. Norton.

Haley, J. (1976). *Problem-solving therapy.* New York: Harper & Row.

Haley, J. (1984). *Ordeal therapy.* San Francisco: Jossey-Bass.

Haley, J. (Ed.). (1985). *Conversations with Milton H. Erickson, M.D., vol. 1: Changing individuals.* Washington, DC: Triangle.

Haley, J. (1990). *Strategies of psychotherapy* (2nd ed.). Rockville, MD: Triangle Press.

Hayward, J. (1987). *Shifting worlds, changing minds.* Boston: Shambhala.

Hilgard, E. (1973). A neodissociation interpretation of pain reduction in hypnosis. *Psychological Review, 80,* 396–411.

Hoff, B. (1983). *The tao of Pooh.* New York: Viking.

Johnson, M. K., Foley, M. A., Suengas, A. G., & Raye, C. L. (1988). Phenomenal characteristics of memories for perceived and imagined autobiographical events. *Journal of Experimental Psychology: General, 117,* 371–376.

Keeney, B. P. (1983). *Aesthetics of change.* New York: Guilford.

Kirsch, I. (1990). *Changing expectations.* Pacific Grove, CA: Brooks/Cole.

Kirsch, I. (Ed.). (1999). *How expectancies shape experience.* Washington, DC: American Psychological Association.

Loftus, E. F. (1993). The reality of repressed memories. *American Psychologist, 48*(5), 518–537.

Loftus, E. F., & Ketcham, K. (1994). *The myth of repressed memory: False memories and allegations of sexual abuse.* New York: St. Martin's Press.

Lynn, S. J., & Rhue, J. W. (Eds.). (1994). *Dissociation: Clinical and theoretical perspectives.* New York: Guilford.

Lynn, S. J., Rhue, J. W., Myers, B. P., & Weekes, J. R. (1994). Pseudomemory in hypnotized and simulating subjects. *International Journal of Clinical and Experimental Hypnosis, 42*(3), 118–129.

Madanes, C. (1984). *Behind the one-way mirror.* San Francisco: Jossey-Bass.

Malanowski, J. (1999, October 24). Shifting from blood and guts to hearts and brains. *The New York Times,* AR15, AR26.

Matthews, B. (1985). A cybernetic model of Ericksonian hypnotherapy: One hand draws the other. In S. R. Lankton (Ed.), *Ericksonian monographs, 1: Elements and dimensions of an Ericksonian approach* (pp. 42–60). New York: Brunner/Mazel.

Milne, A. A. (1985). *The world of Pooh.* New York: E. P. Dutton.

Nolan, T. (1996). Liner notes for *The Best of Bill Evans Live* [compact disk]. New York: Verve.

Ofshe, R., & Watters, E. (1994). *Making monsters: False memories, psychotherapy, and sexual hysteria.* New York: Charles Scribner's Sons.

O'Hanlon, W. H., & Martin, M. (1992). *Solution-oriented hypnosis: An Ericksonian approach.* New York: W. W. Norton.

O'Hanlon, B., & Wilk, J. (1987). *Shifting contexts: The generation of effective psychotherapy.* New York: Guilford.

Oxenhandler, N. (1996, Feb. 19). The eros of parenthood: Not touching children can also be a crime. *The New Yorker,* 47–49.

Pope, K. S. (1996). Memory, abuse, and science: Questioning claims about the false memory syndrome epidemic. *American Psychologist, 51,* 957–974.

Rambo, W. C. (1999). *Fathers who molest their sons and daughters: An inquiry into understanding.* Unpublished doctoral dissertation, NSU, Fort Lauderdale.

Reviere, S. L. (1996). *Memory of childhood trauma: A clinician's guide to the literature.* New York: Guilford.

Roscoe, S. (1996). *Mind-body conversations: Hypnosis, meditation, and oral poetry.* Unpublished doctoral dissertation, NSU, Fort Lauderdale.

Rossi, E. L. (Ed.). (1980). *The collected papers of Milton H. Erickson on hypnosis, vol. 4.* New York: Irvington.

Schacter, D. L. (1996). *Searching for memory: The brain, the mind, and the past.* New York: Basic.

Selvini Palazzoli, M., Boscolo, L., Cecchin, G. & Prata, G. (1978). *Paradox and counterparadox.* New York: Jason Aronson.

Spanos, N. P., Menary, E., Gabora, N. J., DuBreuil, S. C., & Dewhirst, B. (1991). Secondary identity enactments during hypnotic past-life regression: A sociocognitive perspective. *Journal of Personality and Social Psychology, 61,* 308–320.

Spiegel, D., & Scheflin, A. W. (1994). Dissociated or fabricated?: Psychiatric aspects of repressed memory in criminal and civil cases. *International Journal of Clinical and Experimental Hypnosis, 42,* 411–432.

Stevenson, I. (1994). A case of the psychotherapist's fallacy: Hypnotic regression to "previous lives." *American Journal of Clinical Hypnosis, 36*(3), 188–193.

Terr, L. (1994). *Unchained memories.* New York: Basic.

Thomas, F., & Nelson, L. (Eds.). (1998). *Tales from treating families.* New York: Haworth.

Thomas, L. (1990) *Etcetera, etcetera: Notes of a word-watcher.* New York: Penguin.

Watzlawick, P. (1982). Erickson's contribution to the interactional view of psychotherapy. In J. K. Zeig (Ed.), *Ericksonian approaches to hypnosis and psychotherapy* (pp. 147–154). New York: Brunner/Mazel.

Watzlawick, P. (1984). *The invented reality.* New York: W. W. Norton.

Watzlawick, P., Weakland, J. H., & Fisch, R. (1974). *Change: Principles of problem formation and problem resolution.* New York: W. W. Norton.

Weakland, J. H., Fisch, R., Watzlawick, P., & Bodin, A. (1974). Brief therapy: Focused problem resolution. *Family Process, 13,* 141–168.

Wilk, J. (1985). Ericksonian therapeutic patterns: A pattern which connects. In J. K. Zeig (Ed.), *Ericksonian psychotherapy: Vol. 2. Clinical applications* (pp. 210–233). New York: Brunner/Mazel.

Yapko, M. D. (1990). *Trancework* (2nd ed.). New York: Brunner/Mazel.

Yapko, M. (1993, September/October). The seductions of memory. *Family Therapy Networker,* pp. 31–37.

Yapko, M. (1994). Suggestibility and repressed memories of abuse: Survey of psychotherapists' beliefs. *American Journal of Clinical Hypnosis, 36*(3), 163–171.

Yapko, M. D. (1995). *Essentials of hypnosis.* New York: Brunner/Mazel.

# Index